"For those seriously concerned with preventing heart disease, this is your guide: detailed, current, strongly worded guidelines. Yannios, associate director of critical care and nutritional support at Ellis Hospital in Schenectady, N.Y., isn't interested in cushioning the facts or the remedies in a feel-good framework. . . . His horrifying case stories are successfully designed to propel readers into action, and he backs them up with the grim facts: most Americans already heave well-advanced atherosclerosis by their twenties; low-fat diets 'can actually raise cholesterol and increase risk in certain groups of people'; more than half the people who have heart attacks have total cholesterol levels under 200. So the remedy for those in peril, according to Yannios, takes some real work: assess your own risk; then, with the help of a physician, take advantage of the newest blood tests and make a stringent action plan. Guidelines are set out here involving diet, weight control, exercise, and medication. Yannios doesn't let readers off easily, but that doesn't mean he can't offer realistic help: for instance, practically every cardiac risk factor can be countered by exercise; it just has to be the right type of exercise. Heart disease prevention is among the fastest-advancing medical research areas, with new, often conflicting recommendations being published daily. For those at serious risk, this is an understandable, serious, and worthwhile approach."

—*Kirkus Reviews*

THE
HEART DISEASE
BREAKTHROUGH

The 10-Step Program That Can
Save Your Life

Thomas Yannios, M.D.

John Wiley & Sons, Inc.

New York • Chichester • Weinheim • Brisbane • Singapore • Toronto

Published by John Wiley & Sons, Inc.
Published simultaneously in Canada.

ISBN 0-471-35309-4

Printed in the United States of America
10 9 8 7 6 5 4 3

To my parents,
Susan and Christos Yannios,
for inspiring a humanity strong enough
to withstand the cyborg age

Contents

Preface

Heart disease is not a problem for just a few people. Rather, it is a human condition that starts in childhood and afflicts all of us. And the factors that predispose us to having milder or more severe cases are the product of a complex interaction between genes and behavior.

Doctors and cardiologists no longer issue blanket advice to everyone, because we now know that in preventing heart disease, everyone is different. You can't do anything about your genes, but science has armed us with tremendous power to predict how those genes will affect you, and what lifestyle changes you can make to limit their power to cause disease.

Atherosclerosis will not disappear on its own, and no doctor, however well informed, can make it disappear for you. The earlier you adopt healthy habits, the better—it's easier to melt away plaque in a younger person than it is later on, and habits adopted when you are young will serve for a lifetime. You can also play an essential role by gathering information about yourself that might reveal how susceptible you are to heart disease. Many of the tests described in this book won't even be done unless you ask for them.

Atherosclerosis is closely tied to almost every other aspect of your body's functioning—how you digest food, how and where you store fat, how fast your muscles fire, how quickly your blood clots, how avidly your cells consume sugar, and so on. Taking a magic anticholesterol pill or going on the latest celebrity diet isn't going to change the way your body functions. Instead, you must become an active participant in your health care by arming yourself with the knowledge that will help you give yourself the chance to lead a healthy and active life well into old age.

Acknowledgments

This book is the product of extensive research, ongoing experience with patients, and the educational experiences provided by the American College of Cardiology and the American Heart Association. In particular, the workshops, conferences, and seminars presented by the American College of Cardiology and the Berkeley Heart Lab have given me the opportunity to interact with some of the foremost developers of our new understanding of heart disease. I wish to particularly acknowledge the contributions and guidance by Drs. Robert Superko and Ronald Krauss and their enthusiastic and dedicated teams of researchers and clinical associates. These people are in the forefront of forging the newest concepts of the mechanisms of heart disease and the preventative treatment options these mechanisms imply. In particular, they have been instrumental in uncovering the role of LDL particle types in the process of atherosclerosis and the impact of genetic variations of metabolism on proper nutrition.

A book like this doesn't just magically materialize out of a cloud of esoteric information, however. A highly complex and lengthy original manuscript was transformed into a final version largely through the help of Nick Bakalar, who was able to understand the material and resynthesize it. His accomplishment is very impressive, and I will be forever grateful. And credit is due to my senior editor, Tom Miller, at Wiley, whose determined vision of what this book should be sculpted its final form.

My special thanks to Amy Semerad for her thorough and often frenzied word processing of multiple versions of the text, to Amy Olinsky for the graphics, and to my wife, Edith, for her support through what was at times a monstrous task of organizing a half dozen disparate worlds of science into a coherent picture.

Part One

UNDERSTANDING YOUR RISK FOR HEART DISEASE

1

The Heart Disease Surprise: There Is No Immunity

If you opened this book, you or someone close to you has concerns about heart disease. And you're right to be worried: Heart disease and its related problems will end the lives of more people than all the other diseases in the world combined. One of the reasons is that despite all the talk about this disease, despite all the advice handed out freely by doctors and laymen alike, most people still are unaware of how to avoid it. And avoid it you can. If you are properly armed with the latest information, heart disease is almost completely preventable.

Here's a short quiz to determine how sophisticated your knowledge of heart disease really is. Which of the following statements are true, and which are false?

1. The process of atherosclerosis, which causes heart disease, begins at about the age of forty, so you only have to be careful from then on.

2. The first rule for preventing heart disease, which everyone should follow, is eating a low-fat diet.

3. Thirty minutes of moderate exercise accumulated over the length of the day, every day, will significantly reduce your risk for coronary artery disease.

4. If you keep your cholesterol level below 200, you will be fairly safe from getting a heart attack.

5. There are two different kinds of cholesterol, and you have to know both levels to determine your risk.

Although most people—even sophisticated people who are aware of medical facts—don't know it, every one of these statements is false. In the last few years, research has made substantial progress in uncloaking heart disease's secret code as it applies to each individual. In doing so, we have exposed some myths. Here is the real story:

1. The process of atherosclerosis begins in childhood, and in most Americans it is well advanced by the time they are in their twenties.

2. Low-fat diets can actually raise cholesterol and increase risk in certain groups of people. And a good low-fat diet for one person can actually be harmful for another.

3. Thirty minutes of moderate exercise in several short stretches during the day will do almost nothing at all to decrease your risk of coronary artery disease.

4. Many of the people with the most aggressive heart disease have total cholesterols under 200.

5. There are at least a dozen different kinds of cholesterol particles, and their balance in your blood can be the difference between longevity and an early death from heart disease.

You can prevent heart disease, but what you have to know and do to achieve such safety is dependent on your individual mix of risk factors. You have to know what your risk factors are and what you can do to reduce their power over your life. That's what this book will tell you, and it can make the difference between healthy longevity or early death from heart disease. This book presents for the very first time the newest, cutting-edge information now being taught to doctors; it is information essential to anyone interested in preventing a heart attack or recovering from one. The following story shows how insidious heart disease can be.

There Is No Immunity from Heart Disease

It was a routine evening on the maternity floor. When Dr. Pell, the intern on duty that night, was called to see Beth, it was hard for him to believe anything of great importance was happening.

Probably another restless mom in need of a sleeping pill. But when Dr. Pell greeted her from the doorway, Beth didn't answer. She just lay there, eyes open, then closed, restlessly tossing and turning under the sheets, speaking nonsense, apparently having a bad dream.

Dr. Pell and the nurse who had called him both tried to shake Beth awake, but nothing helped. She placed a blood pressure cuff on Beth's arm and looked up at the intern. "Seventy palp." Her blood pressure had dropped 30 points.

Fortunately, the chief resident was close by. "We can't wake her, and her BP's real low," Pell informed his supervisor, Dr. Fisher. The resident peered at Beth. She took Beth's hand in hers and felt her pulse, touched the fingers of Beth's right hand with her palms, then the other hand. They were cold, the fingers a bluish gray, her eyes rolled back in her head. Beth's breathing was fast but regular, and it sounded normal through a stethoscope. Then the resident's eyebrows arched and she looked up. "She's bleeding. Call Dr. Reynolds. Get the OR ready. Get me a central line and 4 units of blood. She's in shock!"

Life-threatening bleeding is one of the more common of the uncommon complications of childbirth, but as Dr. Fisher scrubbed Beth's chest and shoulder with disinfectant in preparation for placing a catheter in her subclavian vein, she realized she hadn't checked the most obvious thing. With her gloved hand, she threw off the bedsheet covering Beth and parted her thighs. There was no blood! "Hmm. This lady had a natural delivery, so if she were bleeding internally there would be blood. Even a ruptured uterus, and there would be the blood."

While waiting for help to move Beth to the ICU, the residents emptied a bottle of saline through the new catheter, placed a 100 percent oxygen mask on her face, and sent for every blood test they could think of to help make a diagnosis. There was very little time. Beth was dying. There were no clues, no suspicions other than what the three doctors saw right before them: a normal new mother mysteriously rendered senseless and in shock fourteen hours after a normal delivery.

In the ICU, Dr. Fisher, the senior medical ICU resident, the chief medical resident, and Beth's attending obstetrician debated what might be happening. They examined and reexamined her. They were joined by both the pulmonary and the cardiology fellows on call, all of them trying to figure it out. But there was little time for discussion. They put the now unconscious woman on a mechanical ventilator. Another catheter was inserted into the large artery feeding her leg to monitor her blood pressure and oxygen level. And another catheter was inserted through Beth's jugular vein deep into the heart to monitor exactly how effectively the heart was pumping. In an attempt to keep her blood pressure up, they pumped thick, protein-rich fluid into her bloodstream and infused adrenalinelike chemicals to force her arteries to constrict and her heart to pump more strongly.

Senior residents in prestigious teaching hospitals rarely bother to consult with attending physicians in the middle of the night. But I was called. The senior resident wanted someone with more experience, and he sensed the need for a pair of "cold eyes," as he put it, to take control of what had become a confusing and emotionally charged case. I was barraged with information the moment I entered the ICU. I craned my neck to read the X ray one resident held up to the ceiling light; someone rustled EKG paper in my ear. The EKG was okay, but the X ray showed that her lungs, which should have appeared black on the film, were opaque white. Then the ICU resident began his systematic account: No, she wasn't bleeding; no, the EKG was correct—she wasn't having a heart attack; no, she had not become infected during delivery, since she had no fever and her white blood count was normal. And yes, the lungs were providing almost no oxygen to the blood.

Of even greater interest to me was the information we could garner from the catheter in Beth's heart. Here we could measure the circulation pressures in the heart-lung system, gauge the amount of blood expelled by each heartbeat, and sample the blood as it was being ejected from the right ventricle into the lung—before it received any new oxygen from the lung. The right ventricle propels this returning blood into the lungs where it is recharged with oxygen. Then it flows through the left ventricle and into the arteries to bathe the cells of every organ. When the flow is thick and fast, the cells are saturated, and they tap only a small portion of the oxygen flowing by. But when the flow is meager, the cells suck up as much oxygen from the blood as they can, leaving it depleted of oxygen as it returns into the right side of the heart. Even though there was no reason to believe she was in heart failure, her heart wasn't providing enough blood flow to her body. To compound the problem, her lungs were becoming increasingly incapable of recharging the blood with oxygen. Neither her heart nor her lungs were working right. She was in shock.

Fortunately, the role of the lungs could, up to a point, be duplicated by a ventilator. But circumventing the inadequately pumping heart and getting that oxygen to her kidneys, liver, and brain was more problematic. I watched the nurse enter with two bottles of fluid and saw her set the infusion pump to maximum. The OB/GYN resident's first thought was that she had thrown a big blood clot into her lungs. The others had drawn more or less the same conclusion. It was either a large blood clot—that is, a pulmonary embolus—or, even more damaging, a lump of amniotic fluid that, on rare occasions, finds its way into the bloodstream rather than being completely delivered with the baby. Either event is catastrophic because they both physically block the flow of blood and set off a violent inflammatory reaction. The lungs become engulfed, choked with fluid, blocking the diffusion of air into the blood. It's as if the patient were drowning.

We'd induced air pressures into the lungs, which can get transmitted everywhere in unpredictable ways. These pressures can distort the heart catheter readings and can also compress the veins that supply the heart, further blocking blood flow. That's why the doctors believed that the heart was nearly empty, despite the readings we were getting.

I admired the sophisticated reasoning, but I didn't agree. I scrutinized the numbers and matched them against what the residents were doing to reverse the shock. It appeared to me that the lungs weren't the real problem at all; it was the heart. No matter how much blood flowed into it, the left ventricle was unable to expel enough blood. This occurs rarely in pregnant women. For some unknown reason, pregnancy produces a cardiomyopathy where the entire heart muscle becomes profoundly weakened and can't pump blood effectively. To confirm this, I borrowed the ICU resident's calculator and more carefully analyzed the resident's readings. Yes, the heart muscle itself seemed weak.

But we couldn't determine whether we should give more fluid for a blockage in the lung, or more medicine for strengthening the heart's beat. To answer that question we would have to look at the heart itself. An echocardiogram could provide a moving picture of the heart, which would show us one of two things: If the heart was swollen and hardly moving, the diagnosis of a primary heart problem was correct. We would then treat it with the appropriate medication. If it showed a small, hyperactive heart desperately trying to supply a flow of blood to the body, that meant the damaged lungs were obstructing the blood return from the body back into the heart. Then fluids would be the correct treatment. Within an hour, we had our echocardiogram.

Gallerstein, the cardiologist, was annoyed. "No, there's something wrong here. I've got to get a better picture." He repositioned the transducer on Beth's chest.

"The left ventricle's not moving well at all," I concluded, looking at the screen.

"Look again," Gallerstein challenged, with his usual caustic tone and rapid-fire delivery. "Does this lady have coronary artery disease?"

"I doubt it. She's only thirty-five years old!" I reassured him. "Isn't it just the anterior wall that's not moving? Why?" I asked.

"Well," he answered, "if I didn't know better, I'd think I was looking at one of my big MI's upstairs," Gallerstein said, referring to his heart attack patients.

"How often do you see a myopathic ventricle look like this?" I asked.

"You don't. She looks like an MI," Gallerstein shot back. "The heart's not even big." A heart damaged from pregnancy is uniformly weak; all of the walls of its ventricles contract poorly. A heart damaged by a blocked coronary blood vessel will show weak contractions only in the wall of the ventricle supplied by that artery. The latter seemed the case with Beth's heart.

We looked at each other in amazement. "Let's get another EKG now!" I shouted to no one in particular.

No one had thought of repeating Beth's EKG. There was no reason to. But when we did, the second EKG told a radically different story from the first. There in the sections of the EKG that corresponded to the section of the heart that was not moving on the echo screen were the unmistakable traces of an acute infarct. It showed us that at some time between the first EKG and now, Beth had had a massive heart attack that practically paralyzed the left ventricle.

My residents were expecting to see a normal heart. I was expecting a bloated sack, almost uniformly still. But what we were seeing was a large, discrete section of the left ventricular wall not moving as it should. This is the typical picture of an infarcted heart muscle because only the muscle supplied by the clogged artery dies. No wonder Beth remained in shock. To stay alive, Beth needed powerful medications to keep her blood pressure up and make her heart more forcefully squeeze out the blood it contained. But she was in complete heart failure, and now we worried that we'd soon see blockages of her other coronary arteries if this level of stress continued.

Beth did not get better. Her shock state was stabilized, but at a low level of heart performance, and as each day passed, the other organ systems began to show the effects of inadequate blood flow. Even so, she might have made it if pneumonia hadn't invaded her lungs. It was a big infection, raising the demands on her heart and circulation to impossible levels. This time, we could not reverse the shock.

Two weeks after the birth of her son, Beth's husband looked at me, pain on his face. "I want to bring her our son. Can you wake her?" I agreed to stop the infusion of sedatives that had kept Beth mercifully senseless. When they wore off, Beth opened her eyes and gazed randomly around the room. I couldn't tell if she really saw her son, or felt his touch when her husband laid the baby on her chest. Beth died the next day.

This was 1984, when we were just beginning to drag the still cumbersome echocardiogram machines into ICUs to help us discover all sorts of surprises about our patients. Had we never done the echo, Beth's death certificate would have read "cause of death: peripartum cardiomyopathy," the intractable heart failure that rarely and mysteriously accompanies a pregnancy.

The findings at Beth's autopsy were shocking. The major branch of her left coronary artery had a large atherosclerotic plaque with a fresh thrombosis, a blood clot that completely sealed off any blood flow. One expected to find this in a sixty-five-year-old, not a new mother. Her other coronary arteries had smaller but similar lesions. So did her aorta, the big artery that receives all the blood directly from the left ventricle.

I don't know if what he saw on my face was wonderment or horror, but as he was removing his gloves and cleaning up after performing the autopsy, Dr. Bala turned to me. "Oh, yes," he assured me, "we see a lot of this in young people. She's an extreme case because of the infarction, but we see this kind of atherosclerosis all the time at this age." I shook my head, and

Bala patted me on the shoulder. "There's no immunity from heart disease."

The inspiration for this book was born with that statement— that and the horrible image of the cooing baby lying on his dying mother's breast. I scanned my memory of cases: The bicyclist with massive head trauma who mysteriously died in heart failure. The auto mechanic crushed by a car when a jack slipped who died of irreversible cardiac shock. Another postdelivery mother who threw a blood clot to her lung and whose autopsy showed a week-old heart attack.

Heart disease does not begin with chest pain. Even as a teenager growing up in the 1960s, I was aware of what is one of the most famous medical studies of all time, Major William Enos's autopsy examinations of three hundred young soldiers killed in the Korean War. The average age of his soldiers was only twenty-two, yet three-quarters of them had significant atherosclerosis in the arteries of their hearts. A study of Vietnam casualties showed much the same thing, but the atherosclerosis was not as severe or widespread. Was this an indication that the population was adopting healthier lifestyles? One might have hoped so, but a study conducted in the 1990s gave little reason for optimism. This time, young people killed by homicide or accident, men as well as women, were studied in Louisville, Kentucky. The findings were depressing: 80 percent of these young people (their average age was twenty-six) had significant atherosclerotic lesions in their coronary arteries, and one in five had lesions so advanced they blocked more than half of the blood flow through the channel. One in ten had an almost completely blocked artery. These were virtually the same as the findings in Major Enos's study forty years earlier.

We have come to understand that heart disease is more akin to arthritis than it is to pneumonia or peptic ulcer disease. It isn't something that strikes us out of the blue or that is produced exclusively by behavior, in the way lung cancer is caused by smoking. Rather, it is a condition bestowed on us by our genes and is the result of a physiology that actually evolved to *sustain* life in humans. But early man lived under conditions that were quite different from those of men and women entering the twenty-first century. The human being for whom our physiology evolved lived a life of constant motion: chasing animals and being chased by them, dressing and cooking the catch, building and rebuilding shelter, foraging, migrating, fighting. The amount and type of food available was always in precarious balance with need. The things that bring misery and death to modern humans—LDL cholesterol particles, cholesterol receptors, triglycerides, blood-clotting factors, immune scavenger cells—not only helped our ancestors heal their wounds but also allowed them to store food in times of plenty against the inevitable times of scarcity that followed. Times of scarcity—at least for the fortunate—no longer exist. But the physiological mechanisms designed to deal with them live on. This book shows you what you can do about it.

2

Heart Disease
Begins in Childhood

It has long been common knowledge that babies develop accumulations of cholesterol on the walls of their major arteries. These accumulations are contained within the bodies of predatory immune cells that are somehow stimulated to grab particles of cholesterol called low-density lipoproteins (LDLs) and intermediate density lipoproteins (IDLs) circulating in the bloodstream as they light upon the arterial wall. Once captured, the LDL and IDL cholesterol particles remain harmlessly contained within the bodies of these predatory cells.

In their first days of medical school future doctors used to learn about these so called foam cells, named for the foamy accretion of globules of cholesterol particles filling their interiors. Medical students were told they were harmless, for after a few years the cells would just melt away.

All true. But because foam cells in babies are harmless, doctors were thereby enticed to downplay the connection between the subsequent nascent cholesterol collections of older children and clinical heart disease.

But now, large-scale systematic studies document a slow but relentless reappearance of these foam cells as children approach puberty. Two-thirds of fourteen-year-olds have not only these isolated cells. They also have a coalescence of masses of these cells that are mixed with pools of free cholesterol oozing from the ruptured carcasses of foam cells that have died from overeating the LDL particles.

As a child matures, these predatory cells are tricked into capturing more and more cholesterol particles. These foam cells enlarge, and when the cells die, the creamy pools of liberated fat coalesce and begin to form cholesterol plaque. Not every one of

12

these streaks of fat laden with foam cells will evolve into a swollen, hardened protrusion into the channel of an artery nourishing the heart muscle. But the more of these coalescing foam cell pools there are, the more fertile a field for heart disease later in life.

Studies show that 10 to 30 percent of the surface areas of all of the aortas of fifteen-year-old boys and girls are covered with this plaque. By age thirty-five, this growth covers between 20 percent and 50 percent of the surface area of the artery. The coronary arteries, the arteries of the heart muscle itself, show less surface area involvement than in the aorta, but the plaque there grows faster. By the age of thirty-five, 75 percent of men and women have such plaque in their coronary arteries as well as in the aortas.

This bulging collection of fat accruing in the arterial wall acquires a canopy of cells and fibers and then begins to harden. After it hardens, the lesion does not melt as easily, as the cholesterol molecules are not absorbed as readily. The lesion now has form, and as it swells from absorbing more and more cholesterol particles from the circulation, it bulges more and more into the channel of the artery. Then, the stage is set for the final evolution, which occurs when a crack or rupture develops on the artery's surface. This stimulates the blood-clotting system to now amplify the size of a modest lesion by layering clotted blood upon it. From here the lesion may take two paths. It can incrementally progress in a kind of layering process that may take another thirty or forty years, or the bulging cap can mushroom, even rupture, causing a complete or near complete blockage of the artery. These ruptures can occur even in people in their twenties.

The genetic codes that have evolved to make some of the cholesterol particles maximally efficient in transporting the fat in our diet also give those particles the ability to stimulate the formation of the "foam cell" and its subsequent evolution into a cholesterol plaque. Moreover, they make the early plaques more prone to these tiny fissures and ruptures. No one knows for sure why the blood clotting system works with cholesterol in this way—it may be that the clotting system is trying to heal these tiny injuries. In any case, by the age of forty heart disease has silently established itself in almost everyone. And in some, it appears much sooner.

The autopsy studies also show who is at higher risk, because while methodically documenting the extent of atherosclerosis in these young bodies the researchers have also carefully recorded the characteristics of those in whom they found lesions.

Almost everyone knows that certain things increase the risk of heart disease: high "bad" or LDL cholesterol levels, low "good" or HDL cholesterol levels, smoking, high blood pressure, diabetes, being male, obesity, poor diet, and of course, age. These risk factors for heart disease are well established in epidemiological and autopsy studies. Changing a child's diet, for example, can lower LDL cholesterol levels, which can result in a dramatic difference in the production of lesions in the coronary arteries before the age of thirty-five.

Teenagers who are at the higher range of LDL and total cholesterol and the lowest range of HDL cholesterol—especially those who smoke—have more than three times the extent of atherosclerosis in their aortas than their counterparts with low LDL levels and high HDL levels. More than 30 percent of an artery's surface area will be affected. In the next twenty years that involvement rises to 50 percent while kids in the low-risk group expand their lesions to cover almost 20 percent. These findings bring a shudder to every parent of a smoking teenager, but they are exactly what the large epidemiological studies show.

How have we been able to establish that these factors really cause heart disease? Although we can't actually observe the arteries of those with various risk factors to see how many of them develop heart disease, we can track young people by their risk factors and see what happens.

This is exactly what was done with more than 1,300 medical students at Johns Hopkins Medical School. The students were selected in the late 1940s and watched into the 1990s. The results confirmed the implications of these autopsy studies and should put to rest any doubt that the incidence of heart disease is directly connected to the presence of these risk factors at a very early age.

The study focused on one important risk factor: cholesterol. The students were divided into four groups according to their cholesterol levels. The incidence of heart disease decades later increased in direct proportion to each group's initial cholesterol level. The group with the highest initial level had four times the amount of heart disease as the group with the lowest level. In fact, each 36 mgs of increased cholesterol carried more than a 70 percent increased risk for developing heart disease, and a 100 percent increase in the risk of actually having a heart attack. This was independent of any other risk factors.

Thus, if the roots of coronary artery disease actually stretch way back into early childhood, then to prevent the disease this process must be interrupted early in life. This is vital: The earlier intervention begins, the better it works.

Just as those fatty streaks in babies are mysteriously dissolved by unknown natural processes, so too can those later cholesterol accumulations appearing around puberty be dissolved. As the lesions begin to swell and start to acquire their fibrous mantle, their cholesterol can still be reabsorbed, and the lesion made harmless. Even later, as layer upon layer of blood clots add to its threatening growth, the clot itself can be attacked and dissolved. But the longer a lesion is allowed to grow, the harder it is to eliminate.

More than a dozen elaborate medical studies have shown us that when a lesion has finally grown to the point where it obstructs so much blood flow in the coronary artery that the symptoms of heart disease are produced, even the most intense and conscientious lifestyle and diet changes, and the use of cholesterol-lowering medications, result in minute shrinkage of the now resistant lesions. There is still a benefit from these kinds of interventions because they arrest further growth and stabilize the fragile canopy of fibers and cells, which are prone to rupture. But such interventions rarely appreciably shrink such advanced lesions after a person is no longer young.

The most elaborate of these autopsy studies, the PDAY (Pathological Determinates of Atherosclerosis in Youth) study, is still going on and has examined the arteries of more than three thousand young people. Cataloging the incidence, extent, and natural history of atherosclerosis would be enough of an accomplishment, but the real purpose of the study is much more forward looking: to describe the exact relationship of risk factors to the anatomical process of atherosclerosis.

It may seem as if we've already done that, and with respect to smoking, obesity, diabetes, high blood pressure, age, cholesterol levels, even race, we surely have. The problem is that this same research has discovered that these risk factors account for only about 50 percent of the behavior of the pathological atherosclerotic process. And as you're about to see in the next chapter, this same battery of risk factors is a very poor predictor of whether or not symptomatic coronary artery disease will occur in a *specific* person, because everyone has a unique genetic background combined with varied lifestyle and behavioral choices.

The PDAY researchers are now applying the most advanced analytical technology to further refine our picture of the composition of these atherosclerotic lesions and catalog the different types of cholesterol particles that form them. Particularly exciting is the next step being undertaken: determining the relationship between different compositional types of cholesterol particles and the genetic coding variations responsible for those types. The process, which was simplistically seen as resulting from the interaction of a certain cholesterol level with a limited list of risk factors, is now revealed as being radically more complex. The complexity derives from the properties of these compositional particles as they interact with the traditional, established risk factors I've mentioned. Perhaps the most revolutionary aspect of this new concept of atherosclerosis and the coronary artery disease it produces is contained in this word: *particle.*

One of the discoveries these pathological studies have made was that two people with the same cholesterol level (that is to say, the same number of cholesterol *molecules* circulating in their blood) and the same behavioral and environmental risk factors can have very different levels of atherosclerosis in different arteries because of the properties their cholesterol *particles* exhibit. But though these particles are largely influenced by genetics, the genes and what they do can often be switched on and off by behavioral and environmental inputs.

Contrary to common conception, cholesterol molecules are not floating free in the blood, waiting to stick to our arterial walls. Rather, the molecules are bundled into *particles* with many different structures and properties. As you're about to see, it is the nature of these particles that governs how cholesterol behaves.

3

Fatal Markers

A very confident forty-eight-year-old man strode into the hospital that morning. Finally Ken was going to get rid of that annoying lumbar disc. No more back pain. No more canceled vacations. Physical therapy hadn't worked, but now surgery would solve the problem. Then back to marathons and tennis games.

The operation started out normally, but afterward something went terribly wrong. As he woke from the anesthesia, he felt more than the expected pain. Faintly, he felt the cold metal of a stethoscope slide across his back while garbled voices mingled with the whoosh of pressurized oxygen bombarding his face. Everywhere there was sensation: the prickling of needles in his hands and wrists, a blood pressure cuff squeezing his right arm tightly, then loosely, then tightly again. A voice floated numbers across his right ear: "Ninety over sixty. Seventy over forty." He leaned forward, trying to push against the invisible weight crushing his chest. He opened his mouth as wide as it would stretch and filled it with the cool mist flowing from the mask. The air flooded his mouth, his throat, but unnervingly stopped there. He repeatedly wrenched the mask from his face and coughed the red-flecked froth away only to have a hand methodically reposition it each time, tightening the straps, centering the green plastic over the nose and mouth. Air, he craved air!

By the time I arrived, at two in the morning, he was already in the ICU, and as I walked to his room, a nurse slapped an EKG tracing in my hands. "You'll get no sleep tonight," she warned. The tracing showed a very large heart attack across the entire front wall of his left ventricle. I immediately intubated him and put him on a ventilator. Then I threaded a catheter from his jugular into his heart, from which a constant flow of data could guide my administration of powerful drugs that forced his heart to beat strongly enough to sustain his body through the crisis.

Today we have the ability to stop a heart attack dead in its tracks and even reverse it. At the very least, we can minimize the amount of permanently damaged heart muscle. For most patients, this level of aggressiveness is as routine as it seems miraculous. But in Ken's case, it was impossible. All such aggressive options require interfering with the blood's ability to clot, and after spinal surgery, such treatment would very likely have left him half paralyzed from destructive bleeding around his spinal cord.

And so we had to keep him stable until enough time passed to make it safe for coronary bypass surgery, the best hope he had of a decent recovery so long after the actual heart attack. I turned to Ken's chart. As the day shift filtered into the ICU, I finally had the time to find out who my patient was.

I scanned his history. He had no major medical problems, just the escalating annoyance of a ruptured lumbar disc. There were none of the personal risk factors for heart disease except one: His father had suffered the first of four heart attacks at the age of forty-five! Because of this, the medical consultant had checked Ken's blood lipid levels and had had him undergo a stress test, which was negative.

Ken's blood tests weren't particularly revealing: His total cholesterol was 190, HDLs 45 (the "good" cholesterol), giving him a total cholesterol to HDL ratio of 4.2. With these numbers, he was what the National Cholesterol Education Program guidelines would categorize as low risk. The rest of the laboratory results were not reported. Obviously, the doctor doing the report didn't consider them worth mentioning and was satisfied that Ken probably did not inherit the severe problems of his father.

And why not think this? Ken's stress results coincided with the accepted interpretations of his cholesterol numbers, and after all, the probability of inheriting his father's problem was a worrisome but far from inevitable fifty-fifty chance.

I leafed through the pages. There on the last sheet were the actual lab reports. LDL 107, triglyceride 190. There were nuances here that were disturbing. This person was an athlete. Despite his back pain, he managed to train for six- and ten-kilometer races. His HDLs (which rise with such prodigious amounts of exercise), though technically okay, should have been considerably higher than 45. And the triglyceride level of 190, again, not alarming in the context in which it was originally interpreted, signaled to me that something was amiss, especially in light of his father's history.

Before Ken's triple bypass surgery, which was accomplished uneventfully, I made his wife promise to bring him back to my office after he had fully recovered. I kept track of his postoperative progress until he was discharged. Then, three months after his ordeal, Ken returned to my office to have blood drawn for special tests I wanted performed by a laboratory thousands of miles away.

Ken's total cholesterol was below the danger point of 200. Moreover, the "bad" component, the dangerous LDL cholesterol, was only a little above 100. That number is low enough for most physicians to assign a low priority to pursuing aggressive LDL cholesterol reduction as a goal, even for a person with overt heart disease, because in keeping with the common conception of this disease and its interplay of risk factors, this particular patient's quantity of LDL just wouldn't be considered a major culprit in his story.

Thus, I could predict that once his active disease was stabilized by bypass grafts, his treatment would involve using medication to minimize the stresses on his heart and to protect and fortify it against the predictable counterattack of the processes causing his disease in the first place. The processes themselves could neither be visualized nor targeted for therapy. But there really was no mystery here. The special tests I had ordered confirmed my suspicions. Contrary to the first impression, Ken had a collection of fatal genetic markers. He had inherited his father's lethal genes.

There was a lot more to his LDLs than just a low number. The number itself referred to just the aggregate amount of cholesterol contained in all of the LDL particles. It told us nothing about the character of the particles themselves. As we've come to understand, just as there is "good" and "bad" cholesterol, there are many genetically determined LDL particle characteristics crucial in determining risk.

One of these characteristics is the size of the particle itself. Ken's was 253 angstrom units. That measurement placed his LDL well into what is called the subclass B type of LDL. This categorization into subclass A and subclass B, depending on the size and other characteristics of the particle, is an essential concept in understanding heart disease risk, one that we will be referring to throughout this book.

Another test, the Lipoprotein (a) level, was a frightening 95, almost twenty-five times the normal level. (This lipoprotein resembles LDL but has the additional noxious quality of promoting blood clots in the coronary artery.) And he had a very high Apoprotein B level as well.

But cholesterol particles are only half of the heart attack story. Cholesterol needs an accomplice to do its final damage, and that accomplice is the blood clot. A high Lipoprotein (a) level and blood that clots easily is a very bad combination. So I sent yet another blood sample to our own lab and confirmed my worst fears that very day: His common blood clotting factor, fibrinogen, was at the upper limit of normal. LDL subclass B, high Apoprotein B, stratospheric Lipoprotein (a), high fibrinogen: This was a portrait of his disease that at once explained his past and predicted his future. Though the quantity of cholesterol his LDL particles contained was indeed low, the tests showed the particles themselves to have characteristics making them extremely virulent in producing the progressive blockage of Ken's blood vessels. Coursing through his arteries, the multitude of his relatively tiny particles frothed and foamed at the point of any crack or ripple of an arterial wall's lining. Densely contracted, the subclass B particles could cross the imperfect microscopic barriers restraining them and accumulate in the blood vessel walls to a degree far greater than his cholesterol measurement alone would have predicted. And if this weren't enough, the gluelike Lp(a) attached itself to many of these same particles, narrowing Ken's blood vessels so effectively that by the age of forty-eight his arteries were ripe for a heart attack.

More than serving as just a shepherd of LDLs, the Lp(a) possesses a number of chemical lures that it uses to trigger the normal blood clotting factors into action. With the passageway of Ken's artery already narrowed, the mushrooming blood clot, fed by increased amounts of the clotting factor fibrinogen, delivered the final blow and shut off all circulation. The heart muscle, dependent on that blood flow, then died.

In all this, nothing had changed when Ken left the hospital. The same processes would attack his bypass grafts, too. His genetic mix predicted it. And it predicted that the rate of injury might even be faster than in his natural arteries. There was, then, great urgency in the report I sent Ken's doctors.

A week later, Ken's brother came to see me to thank me and vent his own fears about the family risks. George, unlike his brother, who was one year older, had a good forty extra pounds hanging over his belt. I vigorously (and I confess rather undiplomatically) urged George to have some blood tests.

Well, not only did George have a cholesterol of 280 and an HDL of 28, but he had a positive borderline stress test as well! His LDLs, which should be as close to 100 as possible, approached 200, and his triglycerides were 240. George was a metabolic mirror of his brother but without the healthy lifestyle. For the time being at least, he didn't need any special circulating risk-factor testing to confirm he was at high risk for heart disease. The standard risk evaluation he received clearly revealed that.

Instead, he underwent coronary angiography, which showed 50 percent to 60 percent blockages of two of his coronary arteries. This wasn't considered enough to necessitate immediate surgery, but it was certainly a very serious problem that could eventually progress to a heart attack. George needed to make some serious lifestyle changes and start on medications, which his doctors hoped might be able to stop the disease from progressing any further.

A few months later I saw both brothers in my office. Ken's cardiologist had placed him on aspirin and an aggressive exercise program along with a heart slowing drug that would lessen the stresses on his wounded organ. George was another matter. Since his cholesterol was already very high, he was put on a regimen of aspirin and a new drug, Mevacor. With it, his original total cholesterol level had dropped from 280 to 148 and his LDL level from about 200 to 110. He had lost twenty pounds and was regularly walking. But his HDLs were still very low, and his triglycerides had hardly dropped. In fact, his lipid profile wasn't too much different from his brother's original values when he'd had his heart attack.

These two needed further testing and treatment. It was time to have George's LDL subclass and Lipoprotein (a) levels checked. As for Ken, I already knew the depth of his metabolic problem, so I called his doctor and discussed the matter. The doctor didn't understand the implications of the LDL subclass and particle size information, and though he knew about Lipoprotein (a), he thought only exercise would help that. I urged that Ken needed special therapy, and after I sent his doctor some information and copies of studies, he agreed.

Meanwhile, George's tests came back. The results were similar to those of his brother. I called his doctor again and told him so. While the Mevacor lowered the total amount of George's LDL, it did not alter the malignant character of the LDL particles themselves. Both brothers needed a drug that would specifically change this malignant, small, dense LDL particle into a larger, less-active type "A" particle; and in this case, that drug is niacin. The common, everyday B vitamin was probably the key to saving both men's lives, especially since it conveniently lowered Lp(a) levels as well.

Niacin may be common, but it can be a very nasty drug when taken in the amounts required to counter those fatal markers. (See chapter 15 for details.) To avoid its annoying side effects requires diligent prescribing and great patience, since the effective dose often needs to be slowly titrated over many months. And both brothers experienced side effects.

Two years passed. I changed locations and completely lost track of the family. Then an urgent phone call plunged me back into the nightmare of that first night. Ken was dead. He had been carrying his clubs on the golf course when he suddenly collapsed. It was another heart attack; though a small one, it was enough to irritate his heart into lethal ventricular fibrillation. The autopsy showed he had occluded the two-and-a-half-year-old bypass vein graft that should have lasted ten years. He left behind a frantic, terrified family. To his brother, Ken's fate was a glimpse of the future. Ken's grieving wife feared for her eighteen-year-old son and twenty-year-old daughter.

Over those same two years, our understanding of these fatal genetic markers had also evolved. The associated risks were much more certain. I referred George to a lipid specialist in New York City who I knew would be persistent with the right therapies.

We did blood tests on the two children, and the son had the same set of lethal factors carried by both his father and grandfather. He also revealed a new twist to this complicated tale. A borderline fasting blood sugar level led me to test his insulin reaction to a structured intake of sugar. Though no one in his family ever had diabetes, he had the same response to the test a diabetic would. Through a convoluted biochemical mechanism, such insulin levels amplified the effect of every one of his genetic problems. It was the final piece of the puzzle.

So Ken's son entered upon a systematic program that first stressed a careful diet and specifically prescribed amounts of exercise. The exercise prescription was translated into precisely quantified levels of intensity and duration for each of the eight different sports that had ever interested him. No weight gain would be tolerated either.

The expanded testing also showed that the son carried a certain genetic marker that predicted he would see a response to the diet and weight loss interventions. So it would be enough for now to see how long a strictly enforced healthful lifestyle could forestall the need for drug therapy.

Without intervention, the son and his uncle were certain to follow Ken's catastrophic course. There was no gray zone here, and Ken's son was fortunate to know it. Now he could adjust his behavior before forming bad habits and construct a lifestyle that would accommodate his genes.

4

It's Not Just
Your Cholesterol Count
That Matters

Ken and his family are not unusual. Their story reflects the evolution that medicine is undergoing in understanding the process of atherosclerosis and how it proceeds to symptomatic heart disease. Their doctors' effectiveness was limited because they were not up to date on our current understanding of heart disease.

In this chapter, I'm going to show you what we now know happens in the arteries of every human being. This is not just an abstract exercise in esoteric scientific knowledge—it is practical information you need in order to evaluate your own risk for heart disease. This is crucial, because you have to know what your risk factors are in order to influence them. As you will learn, any intervention—medication, exercise, vitamin, or diet—must be specifically matched to the problem it is intended to fix. There is no single solution that applies to everyone.

Any level of cholesterol establishes a certain risk for heart attack, and the higher the level, the higher the risk. If your cholesterol level is 200, and you are forty-five years old, you are part of a population that in the next six years will produce six fatal heart attacks for every hundred people with your level of cholesterol. Your odds are six in one hundred over six years. Relative to someone with a lower cholesterol level, you are more likely to have a heart attack. Of course, this describes only a group and says nothing about you as an individual.

The consistency of the relationship between cholesterol and heart disease has been demonstrated in many studies, producing the almost certain knowledge that cholesterol is a cause of heart disease. This relationship is substantiated when pathologists cut open coronary arteries in an autopsy and see that the blockages of those arteries are largely comprised of cholesterol. As further proof establishing cause and effect, studies have shown that when a group of people given an intervention that reduces their cholesterol are matched against a similar group not given that intervention, the former group has fewer heart attacks. So when looked at from the perspective of the entire population, people like Ken whose cholesterol level is at the low end of the scale supposedly don't have too much to worry about, unless some other risk factor is also present. Obviously, this did not work out for Ken.

HDL and LDL

By the late 1980s, we had refined somewhat the picture of cholesterol as the central risk factor for heart disease and distinguished between the different types of cholesterol. We've separated the total cholesterol number into a "good" component called HDL (high-density lipoprotein) and a "bad" component called LDL (low-density lipoprotein). This LDL cholesterol is the source of the cholesterol that pathologists find in the atherosclerotic lesions.

The vessels where the atherosclerosis does its major damage and produces symptomatic clinical disease are those in the aorta; in the arteries supplying the brain, kidneys, legs, and intestines; and of course, in the coronary arteries supplying the heart muscle itself.

The LDL cholesterol particles float in the bloodstream, constantly trying to enter the cells of the arterial wall through small gaps between those cells. At the same time, the cells try to expel a certain percentage of this cholesterol back into the bloodstream. The higher the concentration of LDL in the blood, the greater the pressure to enter the blood vessel wall and the more stressed the protective expulsive forces within that wall become. In almost everyone there is a net deposition of some cholesterol into the walls of the arteries.

The more cholesterol, the more fat is deposited along your coronaries, and the faster the obstructions to blood flow develop. This is happening to you, no matter how low your cholesterol. But in a person with very low LDL cholesterol levels the process has been considered so gradual that he or she would age and die of something else before suffering from the effects of atherosclerosis.

The other traditional risk factors increase the ability of cholesterol to clog arteries. Smoking, high blood pressure, diabetes, obesity, diets high in fat, and stress all facilitate the cholesterol's passage into the wall of the artery either by damaging the integrity of the cell's barrier, or by raising the concentration of the cholesterol itself. Some do both. But without cholesterol these factors can't cause the atherosclerotic lesions that produce heart disease.

How HDLs and LDLs Function

We know about bad LDLs, which accumulate to form vessel blockages, and the good HDLs, which don't. HDLs help the normal protective mechanisms of the blood vessel wall by scavenging the deposited LDL cholesterol and thrusting it back into the circulation, where it is carried by the HDL particle, now engorged with cholesterol, back to the liver to be metabolized and disposed of. This is called reverse cholesterol transport. This reverse transport can be so effective that it can literally melt those soft cholesterol lesions away.

This is why, just as the LDL level and total cholesterol levels constitute major risk factors, the HDL level provides a negative risk factor. The ratio of the two can be very reliably used to place people into high- or low-risk groups.

With varying degrees of completeness, this scheme has been etched into the neural circuitry of every physician from dermatologists to heart surgeons. This picture, omitting a myriad of details about receptors, cell types, cofactors, chemical balances, and kinetics, leaves us with a single core belief: the higher the "bad" LDL cholesterol, the higher your risk.

This "brute force" concept, that the LDL cholesterol mass or level equals risk, has been very helpful in determining overall medical strategies for attacking the problem in the general population. Lower everyone's LDL cholesterol mass and you reduce the number of people in the general population who will get heart disease. So far as this goes, it works: Large studies have proven it.

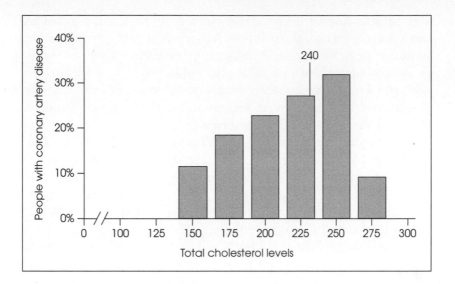

Figure 1

Lowering Cholesterol Doesn't Always Help

But there is a problem with this paradigm. While many lives were definitely being saved by following this rule, too many were not. The contradictions in these studies made a lot of still unsatisfied researchers start looking around for alternative explanations of what exactly was going on in those arteries.

One of the studies that best demonstrated the relationship of cholesterol level to risk for heart disease was the MRFIT study. In Figure 1, the horizontal axis is the cholesterol level and the vertical axis is the percentage of those 350,000 men who died of heart attacks. Clearly, a lot of men died at the lower end of the cholesterol scale. In fact, of the group of men who were at the "lowest" levels of risk, in that they didn't smoke or have high blood pressures, 41 percent who had heart attacks had cholesterol levels below 220, while 24 percent were below 200.

For people who don't already have coronary artery disease or other risk factors, the level of total cholesterol at which standard treatment guidelines advocate automatic, extensive laboratory investigations is 240. In the MRFIT study, 240 misses 47 percent of men who had heart attacks.

The fact is that although heart disease is commonly portrayed as largely caused by high cholesterol, 80 percent of the people who get this disease have the same total and LDL cholesterol levels as those who don't! And should there be any doubt about this, we can turn to the classic heart disease risk study that has served as the foundation of our maturing concepts of risk for this disease, the Framingham Study, done in the town of Framingham, Massachusetts. This, too, is an extensive study of thousands of men and women tracked over time.

This study proved there is an 80 percent overlap of the total cholesterol levels of those who do and do not get heart disease. Total cholesterol isn't the only overlapping classic risk factor. LDL cholesterol, the actual "bad" cholesterol forming atherosclerosis, repeats the pattern. Here it is reconfirmed in a similar survey of the descendants of the original Framingham subjects. Only the people with LDL levels greater than 240 seemed to be in the exclusive "sure to get a heart attack" group. In other studies of the people who developed heart disease, 46 percent had LDL levels below 160—the level at which the National Cholesterol Education Program recommends no further intervention beyond a prudent diet.

So a lot of people with "normal" cholesterol are getting heart disease. Extending this observation is even more telling: Most people getting heart disease have "normal" cholesterols! How is this compatible with the working paradigm of heart disease and the treatment guidelines based upon it? Shouldn't the people developing heart disease be mostly clustered at the high end of the cholesterol scale?

Though a higher percentage of people at the higher levels of cholesterol have heart attacks, there are nevertheless many more people in the general population at the lower levels of cholesterol. So the higher the cholesterol level, the greater the risk. But there are many more people with a cholesterol level of 200 than 300. So though their risk is lower, the absolute number of people having heart attacks will be much higher at cholesterol levels of 200 than the absolute numbers of heart attack victims with cholesterol levels of 300. You see that in Figure 1.

In fact many more people have heart disease and die of heart attacks at the *lower* levels of cholesterol. Dr. Costelli, one of the original Framingham researchers, has long been quite vehement in making fellow doctors aware that the average LDL cholesterol of all people with heart attacks is only 150. That's 10 points below the screening cutoff of established guidelines your doctor might be following when he or she evaluates you. It is important to know what gives heart disease to a person with a "low" or "normal" cholesterol level.

The Group and the Individual

Where your cholesterol level falls puts you into a certain risk group. In that group a certain number of people will develop heart disease over a certain period of time. What this kind of model doesn't do is specify who in any particular group will actually be the unlucky ones. About that, it says nothing at all. The broadly accurate picture in accounting for the behavior of the disease in the entire population does not accurately describe *your* individual risk for accumulating atherosclerosis in your coronary arteries. In fact, it's missing as many people as it's identifying.

Why? If high LDL cholesterol level equals high risk why can't we take this model and accurately apply it to an individual? Why are so many people with "normal" cholesterol levels having heart attacks—even when we eliminate all the other noncholesterol risk factors like smoking and high blood pressure? And why are so many of these people young?

The answer is that the model is really just a sketch, and not a complete script of the drama playing in your arteries. What's really going on has been elucidated only in the past few years. The picture is still far from complete, but enough has been worked out to account for much of the discrepancy between population models and individual circumstances.

A Closer Look at LDL

Let's take a closer look at LDL, shown in Figure 2. It is neither a lump of cholesterol nor an abstract "concentration." It's a particle. This fact determines its behavior as the central risk factor for coronary artery disease. An LDL cholesterol particle is composed mostly of cholesterol but with varying amounts of triglycerides mixed in. Crowning this amalgam is an apoprotein. If the LDL particle can be likened to a cargo ship whose hold carries cholesterol and triglycerides in varying proportions, the apoprotein is the bridge, where the pilot steers the vessel, receives signals

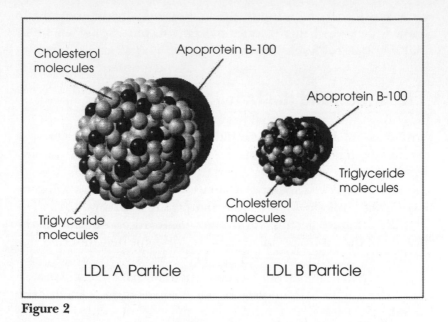

Cholesterol molecules

Apoprotein B-100

Apoprotein B-100

Triglyceride molecules

Cholesterol molecules

Triglyceride molecules

LDL A Particle

LDL B Particle

Figure 2

from the various ports of call, and identifies the ship to others. In the case of the LDL particle, it's called Apoprotein B-100, which will be referred to from now on as Apoprotein B.

Each LDL particle has an Apoprotein B marker, and the number of those Apoprotein B markers very accurately reflects the number of LDL particles in the blood. Why should we care about LDL particles? Until now medicine has been obsessed with the LDL cholesterol *level.* When you receive a cholesterol test result, you get a measure of the milligrams of cholesterol in a given volume of your blood. The lab makes no statement about the number, size, or character of the particles themselves. This was not considered to be particularly helpful information, since according to the model of the disease, it was the abstract, bulk number of LDL cholesterol molecules those particles contained that generated the "pressure" for deposition along the wall of the artery.

Kinds of LDL Particles

But the problem is that not all LDL particles are alike. As Figure 2 shows, there are two families of LDL particles, A and B. In fact, they represent a variable spectrum with radically different levels of malignancy. Seven or more types of LDL particles can actually be differentiated, depending on the methods used to separate and characterize them. Everyone's blood contains this entire range of particles but in proportions that are unique to each individual. Some particles are much more effective at sticking to and penetrating the arterial wall to produce atherosclerotic fat depositions than others, so it is the number and type of these various particles that largely determine how virulent your LDL cholesterol will be.

Variations can be rather dramatic. At the same LDL cholesterol level, regardless of what it is, a person with a bad distribution of LDL particles has a 300 percent greater chance of having heart disease than someone with the "optimal" distribution.

The LDL particles are numbered 1, 2A, 2B, 3A, 3B, 4A, and 4B. Particles with numbers 1 and 2 represent the traditionally conceived LDL particle: a glob of cholesterol attached to an Apoprotein B particle to "steer" it around the circulation. These are the A particles. The far more malignant B particles, 3 and 4, contain less cholesterol because the cholesterol is mixed with variable levels of triglyceride. These particles are smaller and more densely compacted. There is overwhelming evidence that because of the presence of chemical changes induced by triglycerides, the cholesterol in these particles can be more effectively conveyed out of the circulation and into the arterial wall.

There is another purely anatomical reason for the discrepant abilities of the LDL cholesterol particles to penetrate into the arterial wall: The B particles are smaller, as Figure 2 shows, and they can therefore more readily move between the endothelial cells that guard the inner lining of your arteries.

So the big risk factor we must add to LDL cholesterol level is the chemical construction of the LDL particle.

Oxidation

LDL particles slip through the arterial walls and also attach themselves to the walls, damaging the delicate cells upon which they land. They also spear and reel in other potentially damaging cells circulating amid them in the bloodstream and along the arterial wall lining. All of this results from the process of oxidation, and here lies the secret to the extreme virulence of the small, dense LDL particles. They are three times more likely to be oxidized than their larger, less dense counterparts. And oxidization—the same process that causes iron to rust—magnifies their power to accumulate and destroy. The oxidized LDL particle that lights upon a break or irregularity in the lining of the arterial wall, or even one that quietly infiltrates into the wall via those normal gaps in the wall's lining, ignites a reaction that is destined to become an atherosclerotic lesion.

Scavenger Cells and Atherosclerosis

The glob of cholesterol the LDL particle deposits on or in the wall of your artery doesn't just sit there and passively accumulate. It needs anchorage, and as it grows, it needs organization and structure. Ironically, the body's defenses against such invasions will provide this.

When the LDL particle lands within the lining of the blood vessel, it is ingested by the protective predatory scavenger cells that police the immediate environment. These cells are drawn to the globule from both beneath the first layer of the arterial wall and out of the blood streaming by. Once attracted to it, the scavengers swallow the particle. This is the normal mechanism of protection to rid the body of all kinds of microscopic intruders, including infectious agents and debris from trauma. But once this process begins, the scavenger cells find themselves the captives of their quarry. Rather than dispose of the cholesterol, they retain it. And as each cell engulfs more and more particles, it becomes transformed into a bloated reservoir of fat that is now congealed within the cell's protective structure, which is much more resistant to removal than if it were free. These transformed cells are the foam cells, and their formation is the beginning of atherosclerosis.

More Causes of Atherosclerosis

Many other events are also stimulated by the level of oxidization of these LDL particles: The endothelial cells are mutilated if not just killed off, and gaps form where they were. Many of the foam cells reach their capacity limit, rupturing to spill their viscid contents into the core of the growing mass. Other scavenging cells are killed, too, and in their death expel toxic chemicals, which eat away at the arterial wall. So rather than behaving like some quietly accreting amalgam of fat, this growing atherosclerotic lesion begins to resemble an open wound into which are pouring more and more caustic, oxidized LDL particles.

The body strives to heal these wounds. Below the atherosclerotic sore the deeper muscle cells of the arterial wall begin to proliferate, thickening the artery while over the surface grows a delicate canopy of cells and fibers. But the once smooth lining of the arterial channel is forever changed. The usually unobstructed flow of blood must now squeeze past this fat-filled lump, which keeps swelling and expanding as more LDL particles filter into it. This provokes more aberrant structural growth, which even hardens further from calcium accumulations.

Once oxidized, an LDL particle is ten times more likely to attract the cells destined to transmute into foam cells. This is why I refer to these small LDLs as being "malignant." They are thirty times more potent in growing cholesterol plaque than the larger, triglyceride-poor, less-dense LDL A particle.

This depicts a dramatically different model of some of the fundamental forces shaping what is, in effect, not just the development of heart disease but also the aging process itself. These processes affect not only the arteries of the heart but also the arteries of every vital organ in your body.

Medicine for High Cholesterol

One investigation completed in the early 1990s is of particular interest: the Monitored Atherosclerosis Regression Study, or MARS for short. This was an intervention trial with a group of 270 men and women who had coronary artery disease. In this study, the people were divided into two groups. One group was given a low-fat diet; the other was given the same diet plus lovastatin. Lovastatin is a drug that lowers the number of large, less dense LDL A particles, so that the LDL cholesterol level falls, sometimes dramatically. There can be variable effects on other lipids, but the effective therapeutic focus is on large LDL particles.

Here's what they found. The lovastatin lowered the treatment group's LDL cholesterol remarkably, sometimes as low as the 80s. Such levels would lure the vast majority of doctors into feeling any patient would be safe, as far as cholesterol was concerned, from heart disease. But what was lowered were the large, triglyceride-poor LDL particles, not the small, dense, triglyceride-rich LDLs.

The effect of this differential lowering of LDL particles was to impede worsening of the atherosclerosis in the group of patients who had highly advanced, very severe blockages to begin with. These obstructions, which blocked more than half the width of the coronaries, were presumably the older, gradually progressing lesions that responded to lowering the large, slowly accumulating LDL A particles. Overall LDL levels were also lowered the same degree in people who had younger and less severe blockages, but taking lovastatin had absolutely no effect on this group's coronary artery disease. Their lesions didn't shrink. They did just as poorly as the people who received no treatment.

Researchers found out why when they tested for different kinds of cholesterol particles in these patients' blood samples. The tests revealed that the lovastatin treatment didn't affect the more virulent triglyceride-rich cholesterol particles, of which the small dense LDL particles are a major kind. As this and other subsequent studies have shown, it is these particles that seem to be more involved in the development of early or rapidly progressing coronary artery lesions.

Two Families of LDL, Two Kinds of Lesions

There are two families of LDL particles, the large, triglyceride-poor LDL subclass A, and the small, dense, triglyceride-rich subclass B. And there seem to be two courses the atherosclerotic coronary artery lesion can take. Those that progress slowly over decades, and are distinguished by a profusion of "hardening" fibers and calcium, and those that mushroom rapidly and remain soft and prone to rupture and cause a violent artery-blocking reaction.

The MARS study and others like it suggest the relationship that exists between the types of LDL particles and the types of lesions. All atherosclerotic lesions are believed to grow through a series of reactions stimulated by cracks or fissures forming in the

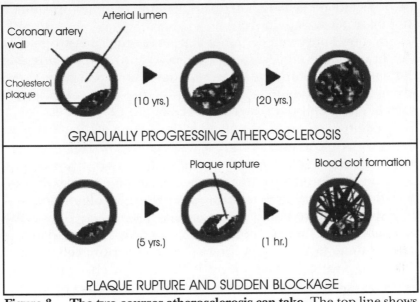

Figure 3. **The two courses atherosclerosis can take.** The top line shows a slowly growing lesion that takes many decades before it blocks the coronary artery. The bottom line depicts the dramatic increase in the level of artery blockage that a small, young lesion can produce after a rupture.

surface of the plaque. When the plaque is composed of relatively stable cholesterol particles, it tends to follow the gradual growing process depicted in the top line of Figure 3. But when the LDL is more reactive in its chemical structure and the lesion more swollen and friable, the reaction to plaque rupture is more violent and complete, as seen in the bottom line of Figure 3.

For years cardiologists have observed, with anguish, that the coronary angiograms they've been doing on their patients couldn't predict where in that coronary arterial tree the next heart attack would come from. What the atherosclerotic obstructions seen on X ray did do was quantify the general severity of the disease and pinpoint the source of many of the patient's chronic symptoms. But the three-quarters-blocked artery torturing the patient with predictable chest pain every time he climbed a flight of stairs wasn't necessarily the artery that would someday completely occlude and try to kill him. It wasn't even the artery that might be responsible for changing the pattern of his chest pain, such as suddenly waking him up at night or creating unprovoked and unpredictable pain.

We now know with certainty that most acute catastrophes of the heart—heart attacks, sudden death, and intense, unstable chest pain—are caused by atherosclerotic lesions that prior to the event occluded less than 50 percent of the open channel, or lumen, of the coronary artery. How can this be?

In more than two-thirds of cases, the sealing off of a coronary artery is not a gradual process, it is a sudden, violent event. Eventually foam cells all disintegrate, spilling their greasy cholesterol content into the center of what has become a heap of stimulated blood vessel muscle cells, scavenger cells, blood clot, and fibrosis that protrudes into the channel of the artery. This is the arterial "plaque," and from here on it can take different paths. It can continue to harden, becoming more and more cellular and fibrotic, growing gradually, layer by layer. Or it can continue to fill up with cholesterol at a rate much faster than this process of "hardening," becoming a soft protrusion into the artery. As with the earlier accumulations of LDL cholesterol, the plaque is in a constant, dynamic equilibrium with the LDLs and the HDLs in the blood that bathe it.

Since the small oxidized LDLs accumulate so much faster, their predominance in the milieu of the growing plaque will not only make it grow more quickly but will also dispose it to becoming a large, soft, fat-filled lesion stabilized by that thin canopy of fibers—something like a tiny cream puff lying in the artery. This is just what has been found when serial angiograms have been used to track the atherosclerotic lesions of people with small, dense LDL. They grow twice as fast in those people as they do in those with the large LDL A particle. And this is where the problem is.

Sudden Events

We know now that those acute cardiac catastrophes are most often caused when one of these soft, cholesterol-filled plaques suddenly ruptures. It is the rupture, more than the size of the lesion, that is so deadly. In fact, the lesions believed to have ruptured are often so small that they can't easily be seen on a prior angiogram at all.

Why does it rupture? Partly because it's so soft. And the softness is in part a result of the rapidity of the cholesterol accumulation. Unlike in more slowly growing lesions, there's a great imbalance between the ballooning, fat-filled center and the hardening outer surface of the plaque.

The chemical nature of the cholesterol itself is also a factor, and the type of cholesterol that is such a problem is exactly the type predominating in those small dense LDLs. In addition, the level of oxidization of the cholesterol plays a big role in continuing to attract those scavenger cells, which can release enzymes that dissolve the stabilizing canopy and rupture the plaque. These mechanisms are closely linked to the type of LDL particles behind the problem.

We don't really know how often these plaques rupture. We don't know why one rupture causes symptoms like chest pain while another causes no symptoms at all. Nor do we know how often symptoms, like an attack of chest pain, are the result of an actual minirupture. We do know that the oxidized LDL particles floating in the bloodstream and not yet deposited in the growing atherosclerotic lesion play an important role in stimulating these events. The event can be anything from a major plaque rupture, which can lead to a heart attack, to a tiny fissuring of the delicate surface of the plaque, which can cause a transient cascade of reactions that temporarily impair blood flow in that region.

We know these LDL particles play an important role because in studies where they have been physically removed from the bloodstream by filtering devices, there is an immediate improvement in heart disease patients' symptoms. The chest pain goes away. Effort tolerances increase. This can't be because of stabilization and regression of their atherosclerosis, since that takes much more time to accomplish.

LDL: Bad News Wherever It Is

So the LDL particle is a menace on both sides of the arterial wall. Inside, it is part of an atherosclerotic lesion; and circulating outside, it is an instigator of instability. This creates a very dangerous synergy between the younger, smaller, softer, atherosclerotic lesions that block less than half of the arterial channel and the level of highly reactive LDL particles, with their retinue of cellular accomplices, freely circulating in the bloodstream.

The occlusion or even partial occlusion of a coronary artery is a violent, dynamic process. With the rupture of the plaque, new culprits other than LDL particles become instantly recruited in the mayhem. The jagged surface of the fissured plaque itself, like torn flesh, stimulates the blood to clot around it. Moreover, the exposed, oxidized cholesterol intensifies this stimulus. Now the circulating blood itself introduces new factors. The various elements of the clotting system come into play. Platelets, the tiny, amorphous cells that stick together to form the initial dam against the flow of blood, adhere to the fissured plaque. They're not only a physical barrier. They also release chemicals that cause the already compromised blood vessel to further constrict and narrow the channel of blood flow. Other chemicals lure clotting factors that, after joining the process, produce a fine, dense web of fibers that traps the passing red blood cells until the entire network forms a dense, impervious clot.

So, depending on the efficiency of the clotting mechanism, the intensity of the inciting physical and chemical triggers, the level of acute constriction of the vessel itself, and the size of the rupture, this collection of cells, fibers, and cholesterol called a plaque will be joined by a blood clot. If the clot is large enough, in minutes it can shut off all blood flow and cause the infarction, or death, of the heart muscle supplied by a blocked coronary, producing a heart attack. In other cases, the ensuing blood clot may just rapidly magnify the original, incomplete blockage, producing a new level of insufficient blood flow. When that occurs, a new or intensified source of chest pain, angina, is created. Pain is the most common response of heart muscle to the insufficient trickle of blood caused by an obstruction.

Risk Factors Beyond Cholesterol

The efficiency of the platelets is a risk factor for heart disease, especially to those people who are known to have atherosclerotic lesions. This is why aspirin, which profoundly impairs this efficiency, has become one of the most miraculously cost-effective lifesavers in history.

It is also why the American College of Cardiology has listed on the official list of risk factors fibrinogen—the substance that transforms itself into the delicate strands of that lethal, blood-trapping web. The more circulating fibrinogen there is, the more readily that web materializes. Therefore, even a high normal fibrinogen level in the blood is a major risk factor.

Two more very potent factors also can influence this clotting phenomenon. In addition to the mechanisms of clotting, the blood contains a mechanism to dissolve clots. Any irregularity of blood flow can trigger clotting: turbulence, partial obstructions, slowing, pooling, and stagnation, especially in sluggishly flowing veins. So the body had to develop a circulating mechanism to dissolve these nascent clots before they become set and immobile. It's called intrinsic fibrinolysis: *intrinsic* meaning naturally occurring in the body; *fibrinolysis* meaning the dissolution of fibrin, the strands of that web formed from fibrinogen.

As we'll see later, the balance between how much fibrin is created from fibrinogen and its dissolution by the fibrinolysis mechanism is another part of the atherosclerosis story. You can profoundly reduce your risk for heart disease by turbocharging the clot-dissolution mechanism. This is a very powerful and elegantly natural way to protect against heart disease. In fact, it is this mechanism that doctors try to reproduce in a person with a fresh heart attack: They inject a fibrinolytic drug to dissolve the clot blocking the coronary.

In one-third of people who go on to develop coronary artery disease, a very nasty form of LDL throws a monkey wrench into this natural balance between forming and dissolving blood clots. It is called Lipoprotein (a), or Lp(a) for short. This is an LDL molecule, complete with its typical identifying Apoprotein B protein, but it also carries another protein called Apoprotein a. This protein inhibits the clot-dissolving process. Like the small dense LDL particle, Lp(a) has a greatly enhanced affinity for accumulation in atherosclerotic lesions. Thus, it presents a double risk. It accumulates rapidly in the plaque then helps the blood clot formation when the plaque ruptures.

As might be expected, this form of LDL has been found to be particularly destructive in people who are extremely dependent upon the ability of the blood to rapidly dissolve spontaneously occurring clots. These are people who have recently had new coronary or other arterial bypass grafts put in, or who have had their atherosclerotic blockages "blasted" away by angioplasty. In these people, the great risk is that new clots will form in the very vulnerable, imperfect new channels of blood flow, and in fact Lp(a) levels have been found to be powerful predictors of the risk for new occlusions in these vulnerable patients.

The last major actor in this drama in your bloodstream is homocysteine. When found in abnormally high levels, this amino acid also promotes clotting, and it has been implicated as a serious risk factor for clotting not just in the coronaries but also in the veins and arteries of the legs and the carotid arteries feeding the brain. Though elevated in only 1 percent of the general population, it is elevated in one-fifth of heart disease patients and one-third of patients with peripheral vascular disease.

As might be expected, high fibrinogen levels and high homocysteine levels create a synergistic threat. As with Lp(a), homocysteine is considered particularly threatening in that same group of recently revascularized patients.

Fissured plaque . . . Plaque rupture . . . Fifty percent lesions . . . LDL particle size, LDL subclass, Lp(a), fibrinogen, Apoprotein B, homocysteine, oxidation . . . These terms are largely absent from the popular discussion of heart disease and probably have never been mentioned by your doctor. But they are essential in understanding heart disease and its prevention.

We've expanded the number of metabolic risk factors considerably. But there are certain behavioral interventions that serve as the foundation for modification of most, but not all, of the components of individual risk. And there is a much greater degree of precision required in matching the intervention, especially in the case of drugs, to the treatment objective. In the following chapters, we will focus on exactly how to go about identifying which of these risks are relevant to you, what your goals should be for every risk factor you have, and how to achieve those goals.

5

Test Your Own Risk: A Quiz

The atherosclerotic process revolves around the LDL cholesterol particle. LDL delivers cholesterol to the arterial wall, providing the stuff of coronary artery disease. This simplified model—"cholesterol level equals risk"—contains at least a kernel of truth. The self-test that follows—the one used by the American College of Cardiology to quickly estimate the risk of heart disease—is derived from a very sophisticated integration of the statistics generated by the large population studies, but it still includes only a few factors: cholesterol, age, sex, blood pressure, and the presence or absence of certain disorders.

This first test determines your broad risk context—that is, you'll see where on the population scale your standard risk factors place you. Add up the points associated with each risk. After you take this test, you'll have one idea of your risk. Then I'll show you how adding in more factors can sharpen the estimate—and may provide some shockingly different results.

1.   The first risk factor is age. This is where the model factors in the head start men have over women in developing coronary artery disease. The scale begins at 30, so if you are younger, use 30.

Age

Women				Men			
Age (years)	Pts	Age (years)	Pts	Age (years)	Pts	Age (years)	Pts
30	-12	41	1	30	-2	48–49	9
31	-11	42–43	2	31	-1	50–51	10
32	-9	44	3	32–33	0	52–54	11
33	-8	45–46	4	34	1	55–56	12
34	-6	47–48	5	35–36	2	57–59	13
35	-5	49–50	6	37–38	3	60–61	14
36	-4	51–52	7	39	4	62–64	15
37	-3	53–55	8	40–41	5	65–67	16
38	-2	56–60	9	42–43	6	68–70	17
39	-1	61–67	10	44–45	7	71–73	18
40	0	68–74	11	46–47	8	74	19

2. Your *total* cholesterol level in (mg/dl).

Total Cholesterol

Mg/dl	Pts	Mg/dl	Pts
139–151	-3	220–239	2
152–166	-2	240–262	3
167–182	-1	263–288	4
183–199	0	289–315	5
200–219	1	316–330	6

3. Your HDL level (high-density lipoprotein) given in units of milligrams per deciliter or (mg/dl).

HDL Cholesterol

Mg/dl	Pts	Mg/dl	Pts
25–26	7	51–55	-1
27–29	6	56–60	-2
30–32	5	61–66	-3
33–35	4	67–73	-4
36–38	3	74–80	-5
39–42	2	81–87	-6
43–46	1	88–96	-7
47–50	0		

4.   Here you need the first (higher) number of your blood pressure, called the systolic blood pressure.

Systolic Blood Pressure

mm Hg	Pts
98–104	–2
105–112	–1
113–120	0
121–129	1
130–139	2
140–149	3
150–160	4
161–172	5
173–185	6

5.   Do you smoke? If yes, add 4 points.

6.   Are you diabetic? If yes, and you're male, add 3 points. If female, add 6 points.

7.   If you've had an electrocardiogram, were you told it showed an enlarged heart? If yes, add 9 points.

Now add up all of your points and look up your risk over the next ten years.

Probability

Pts.	10-year	Pts.	10-year	Pts.	10-year
<1	<1%	12	7%	23	23%
2	1%	13	8%	24	25%
3	2%	14	9%	25	27%
4	2%	15	10%	26	29%
5	3%	16	12%	27	31%
6	3%	17	13%	28	33%
7	4%	18	14%	29	36%
8	4%	19	16%	30	38%
9	4%	20	18%	31	40%
10	6%	21	19%	32	42%
11	6%	22	21%		

For comparison to other groups of people:

Probability
(average 10-year risk for all people in age group)

Age (years)	Women	Men
30–34	<1%	3%
35–39	<1%	5%
40–44	2%	6%
45–49	5%	10%
50–54	8%	14%
55–59	12%	16%
60–64	13%	21%
65–69	9%	30%
70–74	12%	24%

Now you've calculated your risk in the standard way. Here's how that risk can change when we add in more factors. Let's use a theoretical forty-five-year-old Mr. Average. That means he has a

Total cholesterol of 207: 1 point

HDL cholesterol of 42: 2 points

Blood pressure 130/80: 2 points

Giving him the benefit of the doubt: no smoking, diabetes, and a normal EKG

Age 45: 7 points

Total: 12 points

From the chart, his 10-year risk is: 7%

This means Mr. Average is part of a group of a hundred people, seven of whom will have a heart attack in the next ten years. Not bad odds. I certainly would feel safe if I had that kind of risk.

Now let's see what the underlying risk factors do to those odds. There's nothing about what Mr. Average has listed as risk factors that couldn't be hiding any or all of the following risks:

1. Unfavorable LDL particle size $3 \times 7\% = 21\%$ risk

2. Unfavorable HDL particle
   distribution $3 \times 7\% = 21\%$ risk

3. Unfavorable LDL particle variant $3 \times 7\% = 21\%$ risk

4. High blood-clotting factor
   concentration $1.2 \times 7\% = 8.4\%$ risk

For the sake of illustration, let's say after following the self-assessment process described in later sections of this book, Mr. Average finds he has two more risk factors, a combination of No. 1 and No. 2. This increases Mr. Average's risk by three times three, transforming a 7 percent risk into a 63 percent risk. He now realizes he has a two-out-of-three chance to develop coronary artery disease by the age of fifty-five compared to a person who does not have those additional risk factors.

We've taken our Mr. Average and we've honed in on his chances of being one of those seven in his peer group of a hundred people. Of course, a 63 percent risk isn't 100 percent, and even a 100 percent risk is still theoretical, not a certainty. But for most people it is certain enough to make them want to do something to counter it.

Part Two

THE HEART DISEASE PREVENTION PROGRAM FOR YOUR TYPE

6

Step One:
Get All Your Blood Tests—
Not Just Total Cholesterol

You can eat right, exercise, lose weight, and avoid smoking, but you can't change your genes—if you have a family history of heart disease, your risk is as much as five times greater than for somebody with "clean genes."

In the early 1990s, an ambitious group of researchers studied more than 1,200 Mexican Americans from forty-two different families to examine the variable effects of behavior, family environment, and genetics on an array of risk factors for heart disease. They scrutinized what these people ate, how much they exercised, and which parts of their bodies had excess fat. Then they considered an exhaustive list of atherosclerosis risk factors. They found that the effect of genetics was three times as powerful as the effects of lifestyle and environment. In fact, the nongenetic factors like diet, exercise, smoking, and the like could only account for at most 15 percent of the variability in any risk factor. A number of similar studies ranging across the nation from Utah, to Iowa, to Michigan, to Ohio have shown the same kind of genetic power.

Behavioral and environmental factors accounted for only 15 percent of the variability of all these risk factors while genetics accounted for 45 percent. Let's look at an example. The average diet of this Mexican population was composed of about half carbohydrate and about a third fat. The effect of diet on HDL levels was about 1 percent. But the effect of genes was 30 percent to 46 percent. In other words, those who were leading healthy lifestyles—even if they had the wrong genes—were hardly better off than those who weren't.

But this is not a reason to retreat into fatalism. It is important to understand that these studies did not determine how that genetic effect translated into actual heart disease. That is a different issue.

Lifestyle factors account for 15 percent of the variability of risk factors, while 45 percent were genetic. That left 40 percent of influences unaccounted for. So what you do with—or to—your body is still very important, more important than that 15 percent might imply. The design of the study couldn't pinpoint the full magnitude of behavior on risk.

We are each born with a genetic potential for developing heart disease, some of us very great, some quite small, most somewhere in between. To limit the potential for disease our genes have given us, we need to know what genes are involved and what we can do to minimize their effect.

We are at the very early stages of such knowledge, but already it is clear that most medical conditions are the result of an interaction between multiple genes and environment. This is why some people can exist on steak and eggs and never worry about the plaques in their arteries while there are competitive athletes on careful diets who die of heart attacks.

Our quality of life depends on how effectively we nurture the desirable traits we were born with and suppress those that are threats. Success in this requires a detailed, comprehensive, individual analysis of as many of the relevant genes or their markers as possible. Any intervention must be carefully matched to the individual's particular panoply of genetic susceptibilities.

This genetic connection is clinically most evident in people developing heart disease before age sixty.

The medical geneticist Jacques Genest led a group that examined people with coronary artery disease and compared them to a matched group of descendants of the original Framingham Study. They found that the average total cholesterol of the people with heart disease was actually 20 points lower than the healthy controls.

Yet beneath these numbers was a swarm of genetic problems carrying these people to early heart disease. Seventy-six percent of the heart disease group had a genetically linked problem revealed by more detailed laboratory testing, and almost all of these had more than one. Two-thirds of the families showed evidence of transmission to children of one or more of the genetic problems present in the parents.

Genest found an isolated elevation of LDL cholesterol in only 11 percent of his patients. There were four times as many men with profound reductions of protective HDL levels as there were those who had high LDL levels. The other problems that predominated were elevated levels of triglycerides, Lp(a), homocysteine, and the numbers of the LDL particles, rather than the cholesterol mass in the blood.

There was a particularly common triad of abnormalities in a large plurality of heart disease patients: About 50 percent of men and 30 percent of women who develop coronary artery disease have low or low-normal HDL levels, high or high-normal triglycerides levels, and small, dense triglyceride-rich LDL particles.

The standard test for *total* cholesterol reveals only one or two genetic disorders. If you expand your list of tests to LDL cholesterol, HDL cholesterol, and triglyceride levels, then three genetic problems can now be identified. Together, these factors target only about 20 percent of all coronary artery disease patients.

Of the remaining 80 percent, very few of these traits are determined by a single gene. The stratospheric LDL cholesterol levels of a disorder like inherited (familial) hypercholesterolemia, for instance, can be the result of dozens of different genes.

The number you see on your laboratory report for any particular risk factor derives from complex interrelationships between your genes and your behavior: your hormone mix; the amount and type of calories, vitamins, and minerals you consume; the intensity of your metabolism; your weight; the medicines you take; and many other environmental and metabolic factors. But once your genetic traits are revealed, you can change your lifestyle to minimize the expression of those traits, and if necessary, select the treatments that specifically target them.

Today we know that there are many genetic variations that either contribute to these risk factors or constitute risks in themselves. While many have been identified, translating this knowledge into clinically usable tools is a very slow process. Though we know where they are, practically speaking most of these genes can't actually be tested for. But we can easily establish the presence of many of the major markers representing the end products of the activities of these genes. These markers provide a window through which we can see the inherited propensities of any person's metabolism. The standard cholesterol test picks up only four of these markers. Here they are, listed with the disorders they can detect.

Test: Total cholesterol and/or LDL cholesterol

Disorder Name: Familial hypercholesterolemia or FH (extremely high LDL cholesterol)

This disorder is listed first because anyone with LDL levels greater than 250, which is about twice what any genetically "uninfluenced" person should be, has an inherited condition that almost guarantees an early heart attack. The average man so afflicted will usually have a heart attack by age forty-five, a woman by fifty-five. It is found in about 3 percent of people developing heart disease and in only one person in five hundred in the general population. If you have it, more than half of your children can be expected to inherit this problem.

Tests: Total cholesterol or LDL cholesterol and triglycerides

Disorder Name: Familial combined hyperlipidemia or FCH (extremely high LDL cholesterol and triglycerides)

This is another disorder that can be picked up by routine blood lipid tests. In this case, LDL and triglyceride levels may be very high. It is the result of a complex amalgam of genetic variations that frequently cause an overlap of this disorder with many of the other disorders listed later involving HDL and LDL particle type. Twenty percent of coronary artery disease patients have it.

Often only one component is elevated. Medications, diet, exercise, and weight can significantly modulate marker levels, so the problem can be missed unless an overlapping disorder (see following tests) is also picked up on testing. More than half of your offspring can be expected to inherit this problem.

Test: Triglycerides

Disorder Name: Hypertriglyceridemia (high triglycerides)

This marks a number of different disorders. Triglyceride levels greater than 1,000 represent a specific medical problem because the blood literally sludges. Isolated elevations of triglycerides at this level are usually secondary to genetic defects not commonly tested for in themselves. Triglyceride levels in the low 100s range are usually not a problem in themselves but are a manifestation of diabetes or another, much more malignant underlying problem involving LDL particles. Elevations of this magnitude should trigger further testing.

Test: HDL cholesterol

Disorder Name: Low HDL or hypoalphalipoproteinemia (Hypo A)

Levels of HDL cholesterol below 29 in men and 38 in women carry a 200 to 300 percent increased risk of coronary artery disease. Fifty percent or more of offspring will inherit it. The "pure" condition often isn't associated with any other genetic condition. It can be discovered by the HDL test, but can be confirmed only with the Apoprotein A1 test, which actually counts the number of HDL particles, unlike the ordinary HDL cholesterol test, which measures the total amount of cholesterol in the HDL particles.

More often, a low HDL is *not* caused by this genetic condition. Rather it is a secondary problem linked to a bad lifestyle or to an abnormal triglyceride elevation and/or LDL particle metabolism as in the LDL subclass B state.

These four genetic problems, which are picked up on the standard, comprehensive "lipid panel," represent about 20 percent of the patients who develop coronary artery disease. But here are some further markers we now know about. All of these require special tests, but the tests can be fairly easily done if you make a point of asking for them.

Test: LDL subclass and LDL particle size, Apoprotein B

Disorder Name: LDL subclass B, or small LDL, or atherogenic lipoprotein profile (ALP)

This disorder afflicts 50 percent of heart disease patients, 35 percent of the normal male population, 12 percent of normal premenopausal females, and 25 percent of normal post-menopausal females. It carries a 300 to 400 percent risk of disease and is the product of multiple gene disorders. Along with elevated LDL cholesterol levels, ALP is the biggest cause of heart disease.

The small, dense LDL particle is associated with low HDL levels, total cholesterol/HDL ratios greater than 4, and relative elevations of triglycerides.

This disorder is also associated with overt or latent non-insulin dependent (or adult onset) diabetes, high normal fasting blood sugar and insulin levels, and prolonged elevations of triglyceride levels after a test meal—"sludgy blood." As with the other disorders, inheritance is about 50 percent.

The Apoprotein B test gives more accurate *circumstantial* evidence about the presence of small, dense LDL particles. While the subclass B test actually measures the size and size distribution of the particles—parameters that define the LDL subclass—the Apoprotein B test measures the *number* of particles.

High Apoprotein B tests in relation to any given LDL cholesterol levels strongly imply subclass B. When an Apoprotein B level is divided by the LDL cholesterol level to yield a value greater than 1.1, subclass B is almost certain.

Test: HDL subclass

Disorder Name: Poor HDL subclass distribution—low HDL2

Like LDL particles, HDL particles are divided by size and density. There are five different types: two kinds of HDL2, a and b; and three kinds of HDL3, a, b, and c. HDL2 particles carry away the cholesterol for disposal. Elevated levels of certain kinds of HDL3 particles reflect abnormally increased triglyceride content of the HDL particle. This alteration renders this potentially potent protection factor almost useless as a cholesterol scavenger. High HDL 3b complements the increased virulence of the high triglyceride-containing LDL subclass B particles.

High HDL2 levels, especially HDL2b, convey more than twice the protection factor of high HDL3 levels. It's especially important to know this ratio when total HDL cholesterol levels hover around the "average" range, especially if you are working hard to raise them to that level. A high HDL2 level can convert a mediocre total HDL level into a significantly negative risk factor by amplifying its biological potency as a cholesterol scavenger.

Test: Apoprotein E Isoform

Disorder Name: Apoprotein E allele associated risk

This is an actual test of the gene determining the activity of the LDL receptor that attaches to the apoproteins found on various lipid particles. The Apoprotein E structure results from the pair of genes coding for it. There are four variants of this gene, each variant being an allele, one gene coming from each parent. The Apoprotein E structure will determine how LDL particles are cleared from the bloodstream and how diet will affect this clearance.

These genes can combine in six different pairs. Each implies a different risk for heart disease and is associated with different levels of LDL and, in some cases, triglycerides. This is a universally applicable test, since everyone has Apoprotein E receptors, and it can affect heart disease risk by 30 to 40 percent. Most important, it predicts for many people how they will respond to diet changes. (See chapter 12.)

Test: Lp(a)

Disorder Name: High Lipoprotein A or Lp(a)

Lp(a) is an LDL particle with an extra protein called Apoprotein a attached to it. Its presence in the blood can interfere with normal clotting dynamics and promote clotting around atherosclerotic plaques. It also more readily oxidizes and migrates into the arterial wall than even the small dense LDL particle.

One-third of coronary artery disease patients have elevated Lp(a), and such elevations carry a 250 to 300 percent increased risk. The risk is amplified by the presence of high LDL cholesterol levels, LDL subclass B state, elevated homocysteine, and fibrinogen levels.

An Lp(a) level above 20 indicates a risk factor, and a level of 30 in some populations is equivalent to the danger of a total cholesterol of 240! It is also a factor particularly threatening to people who have recently had their coronaries opened by invasive procedures like angioplasty, the opening of a blocked coronary artery by the inflation of a balloon threaded into the blockage.

Forcing an artery open like this, while restoring blood flow, also damages the already injured arterial inner wall. This makes the artery particularly susceptible to reobstruction by blood clots.

About one-half of your descendants will inherit this problem. Its presence cannot be predicted by any other lipid tests.

Tests: Fasting blood sugar, fasting insulin level, two-hour postprandial blood sugar or insulin level, glucose tolerance test, hemoglobin A1C level

Disorder Name: Non-insulin-dependent (adult onset) diabetes

Often the first sign of diabetes is a heart attack. The cheapest and easiest test of all is a fasting blood sugar. You can even do it at home. A significant percentage of people who hover near the upper limit of the normal range above 110 mg/dl have a genetic susceptibility for diabetes. If your fasting blood sugar is consistently on the high side of normal, a stepwise investigation is needed to unmask the underlying condition. The tests are easy to get, though some are quite involved, and they will confirm or deny the suspicion. Diabetes is linked to LDL subclass B, high triglycerides, low HDL, high fibrinogen, and a range of other not as easily measurable abnormalities that so strongly predispose to atherosclerosis formation that this risk complex has been termed the cardiovascular dysmetabolic syndrome.

Fasting blood sugar is a very insensitive marker, so if there is any kind of diabetes in any immediate family member up through your grandparents, a very easy and much more sensitive screening test is a blood sugar level taken two hours after eating a standardized amount of carbohydrate. Adding an insulin level to this increases accuracy even more. So don't be lulled into complacency if your blood sugar results are "normal." Being in the high range of normal, especially with a family member with diabetes or early heart disease, requires more investigation.

Test: Homocysteine level

Disorder Name: Homocysteinemia (high homocysteine levels)

Homocysteine is an amino acid. An aberration of both genes controlling its metabolism results in a well-known lethal disease found in children. When only one of the genes is affected, the condition called homocysteinemia results in a buildup of this amino acid in the blood. This aggravates almost all the mechanisms involved in atherosclerosis. About 20 to 30 percent of people with coronary artery disease have this condition versus 1 percent of the healthy population. It is an even more serious risk factor for symptomatic atherosclerosis involving the arteries of the extremities, affecting 30 percent of such patients. Fasting levels greater than 20 indicate a twofold increase in coronary artery disease risk. There are no associations with any other risk factor values.

In the genetically susceptible person, expression of this genetic disorder is highly dependent on low levels of common B vitamins—folic acid, and to a lesser degree, B_6 and B_{12}. It is a lethal condition with a very simple treatment.

Test: Fibrinogen levels

Disorder Name: High fibrinogen
Fibrinogen circulates in the bloodstream and is transformed into the delicate web of fibers lacing together a blood clot into a solid mass. The normal range of fibrinogen levels is very wide, and any person's level can vary greatly at different times and under different conditions. There are many people, however, who consistently run high levels and whose response to stimuli that normally boost these levels is excessively sensitive. This is a result of genetics and underlying physical conditions such as diabetes, which are known to boost fibrinogen levels.

As one of the primary agents of the clotting mechanism, its presence in elevated quantities is synergistic with the other factors that promote blood clotting: oxidized LDL particles, Lp(a), and homocysteine. People, especially women, at the upper ranges of fibrinogen have a greater than 30 percent increased risk for developing coronary artery disease.

So much for the tests that are relatively easily available. Other tests can reveal further useful information, but these are performed in research labs and are not generally available in commercial versions. I list them below because we can expect access to such tests in the near future, and because these tests demonstrate risk mechanisms that are intimately connected to the actions of those risk factors already listed.

Test: LDL oxidation

Disorder Name: High level of oxidized LDL particles

All LDL particles can be oxidized: large subclass A particles, small dense subclass B particles, and the Lp(a) particles. There are numerous tests employing different markers that can quantify the level of this oxidation in a person's system. This is particularly important when making an intervention to affect LDL oxidation, as it indicates the effectiveness of the intervention. It also allows us to get a better picture of what's going on in the LDL subclass A patient who despite a lower theoretical risk compared to subclass B is developing coronary artery disease. Some people's subclass A LDL particles are very susceptible to oxidation and act more like subclass B particles.

Test: IDL level

Disorder Name: High IDL levels (intermediate-density lipoprotein)

IDL levels supplement LDL subclass information. IDLs are believed to be one of the major reservoirs of the cholesterol that is found in the atherosclerotic lesion. Elevations of IDLs are produced by the same genetic-metabolic forces that produce most of LDL subclass B particles. Prior to the availability of this test, IDL levels were inferred from LDL subclass B information. Many research studies, some of which I will cite in this book, use IDL levels to implicate the same kinds of disease-producing properties ascribed to LDL subclass B particles. Thus they represent, in a sense, a linked risk. Of all the prospective marker tests, IDL levels will probably be available first, and in the very near future.

Test: LPL activity

Disorder Name: Low lipoprotein lipase (LPL) activity

LPL is one of the pivotal enzymes in many of the metabolic pathways that determine relative levels of LDL subclass A and B particles, triglycerides, IDLs and HDLs, and *their* subclasses. Like LDL oxidation, the LPL levels are very responsive to a multitude of interventions, the most commonly mentioned of which is exercise. But diet, weight loss, and various medications and medical conditions such as diabetes also have profound effects on this marker. As such, this test can be used as a direct indicator of the effectiveness of these interventions and could be used, for instance, in determining exactly how much exercise is required for reducing the risk of heart disease.

There are many people with outright genetic deficiencies in LPL activity, which produce malignantly elevated levels of triglycerides and derangements of HDL levels. Measuring it requires having a biopsy. This test is used mostly in research protocols, though it is made available to athletes willing to undergo the inconvenience and expense of the test. A commercial version seems a bit far in the future, but it will be a very important test when it does become available.

Test: Apoprotein C-II

Disorder Name: Apoprotein C-II deficiency
The Apoprotein C-II helps HDL scavenge cholesterol deposited on the arterial wall. A deficiency of it cripples the HDLs' effectiveness. But unlike LPL, this factor circulates in the blood, and we may see a commercially available test for it in the near future. That would be very helpful, since about 12 percent of African Americans suffer serious genetically produced deficiencies, resulting in low HDL levels and high triglyceride levels.

Now you can see the impressive amount of information you can amass about your genetically determined risks for heart disease. But there is still more we know, as the succeeding chapters will show.

7

Step Two: Determine Your Individual Genetic Risk Profile

Don't send your blood out for testing yet. First, let's talk about your family. Family history is a part of every initial medical interview, but it isn't always given the attention it deserves. And nowhere is this kind of information more important than for heart disease.

If you don't know what medical problems your grandparents, parents, brothers, and sisters have had, it is essential to find out. Even the state of your aunts' and uncles' health provides valuable information about the genetic makeup of the family.

Genetics and Risk

Genes are inherited in various complex ways and in various combinations, but most of the coronary artery disease risk factors are dominant genes. So you only need to inherit the gene from one parent for it to be expressed in you. The way the gene is expressed—the degree of severity of disease or disorder it produces, for example—can vary considerably from one person to another, even from one sibling to another. And genes affect the expression of other genes: A person with a gene for high LDL cholesterol may nevertheless have low cholesterol because another gene keeps it low.

How do you put all of this together to steer toward the right evaluation? You obviously can't know whether your deceased father had elevated Lp(a) and low HDL2 levels, or that he got each of one of these traits from a parent, but you can recall the symptomatic problems of each relative, and any clinical diagnoses, like adult onset diabetes.

You can also find heart disease by learning to look for its shadows. Sometimes the blood flow to other parts of the body is affected earlier and more dramatically, creating symptoms—even catastrophes—that don't seem to have anything to do with heart disease. Many patients come to the hospital for surgery because of a threatening problem to an organ system very remote from the heart. Yet the process causing the problem is the same atherosclerosis that affects coronary arteries. They have their surgery without a hitch, then suffer a heart attack two days later, leaving the doctors scratching their heads: "But he didn't have heart disease."

In scrutinizing your family history the clues fall into two categories: First, certain disorders imply severe atherosclerosis, but they just happened to hit another part of the body before becoming evident in the heart:

- Stroke or near stroke (TIAs)
- Peripheral vascular disease (insufficient blood flow to legs, feet, toes, hands, fingers)
- Claudication (recurrent cramping, usually of leg muscles, with exercise)
- Kidney failure
- Bowel or intestinal infarction (complete blockage of blood flow to a part of the intestine)
- Intestinal pain, cramping, or inflammation resulting from lack of blood flow (blood ischemia or incomplete blood flow blockage)
- Aortic aneurysm
- Irregular heart rhythm

Second, certain problems themselves promote the development of heart disease:

- Diabetes
- High blood pressure
- Obesity

Any one of these is a major risk factor. However, they commonly occur together, and when they do, this may be part of an underlying physiologic and metabolic state highly disposed to the development of coronary artery disease. It's easiest to make a list and check off what you know about your family. Here's an example:

Mother's Side	Father's Side
Grandpa? Died age 69	Grandpa—Died accident age 45
Grandma—Died of cancer age 76	Grandma—alive
Mother—No heart disease age 70	Father—chest pain, coronary artery disease, age 59

You and Your Siblings

Brother	*Me*	*Sister*
OK age 37	OK age 45	OK age 40

On your mother's side, there's no evidence of heart disease. On your father's side, there's much more activity. Clearly, there's a problem here: Your father's coronary artery disease at an early age.

This brings us to you and your siblings. Because of the father, all three of you are immediately in a much higher risk category. Since there are probably numerous identifiable genetic problems here, it is fully justifiable now to proceed with an investigation of just what is causing the high risk.

A way to streamline this process is to go right where the problem is, your father. Testing him will uncloak the risks and narrow down the list of tests the three children need. Here are the hypothetical results of your father's tests:

LDL cholesterol of 130

LDL Subclass B (predominance of small, dense LDL particles)

High Lp(a) of 57

Borderline HDL of 38, HDL2 low

Average triglyceride of 120

Negative homocysteine level

Your father has numerous genetic problems: He's an LDL subclass B, he has low HDL2 (the more protective part of the HDL family), and his Lp(a) is high. On the other hand, his LDL is not unusually high for his age, and homocysteine isn't a problem. This means that in addition to a baseline, lipid panel of total cholesterol, LDL cholesterol, and HDL cholesterol and triglycerides, each son and daughter should see if they have inherited the subclass B state and the high Lp(a) by including those tests in their profile. I wouldn't do the HDL subclass test until I knew what the total HDL cholesterol level was.

In this case, each child has inherited the subclass B state, and one also has the high Lp(a). The investigation was streamlined and very economical because we already knew what to look for. In addition to the usual list of conventional risk factors, the LDL subclass B added another major risk factor to the profiles of you and your siblings, and for the child with high Lp(a), two additional major risks.

If the parent with premature coronary artery disease is not available for testing, you should presume the worst and undergo a comprehensive battery of tests.

Suppose you had a grandparent who had heart disease, but your parent escaped. Look for a reason why. Did your grandparent smoke, thereby reinforcing some genetic risk factor and making it more effective in producing disease? Is there a major difference in diet, weight, lifestyle, and exercise level among you, your parent, and your grandparent? Look for things that you know can amplify or attenuate risk. You may be repeating the lifestyle of your grandparent, who had heart disease, rather than that of your parent, who didn't. Evidently, the risk factor or factors your parent inherited are being counteracted. This counteraction could either be something else your parent inherited from your *other* grandparent, who didn't have heart disease, or a lifestyle factor.

A useful project is to take all of this family information, and whatever test results you have from your relatives, and create a genetic tree. This will help organize your own thinking, and it can prove a valuable piece of information for your doctor when

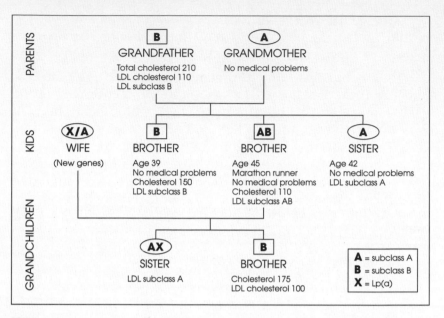

PARENTS

B
GRANDFATHER
Total cholesterol 210
LDL cholesterol 110
LDL subclass B

A
GRANDMOTHER
No medical problems

KIDS

X/A
WIFE
(New genes)

B
BROTHER
Age 39
No medical problems
Cholesterol 150
LDL subclass B

AB
BROTHER
Age 45
Marathon runner
No medical problems
Cholesterol 110
LDL subclass AB

A
SISTER
Age 42
No medical problems
LDL subclass A

GRANDCHILDREN

AX
SISTER
LDL subclass A

B
BROTHER
Cholesterol 175
LDL cholesterol 100

A = subclass A
B = subclass B
X = Lp(a)

Figure 4

you are being evaluated—not just for heart disease, but for any medical problem.

Let's say you wanted to keep track of the LDL subclass B risk in your family. Take a look at this sample family tree in Figure 4.

Here we have a very simple family tree of another family where the grandfather is subclass B and grandmother is subclass A. There are no other abnormalities in the original family. If there were, you could create a symbol for each and place it in the appropriate box or square, as is shown with the newcomer to the scene, the forty-five-year-old brother's wife. Here X means an elevated Lp(a). The children show one of each of the possible LDL subclass patterns consistent with the underlying gene pairing. It's quite possible that the sister will convert to a subclass B after she passes through menopause. The brother, if he ever stops exercising vigorously, would probably also convert to the subclass B state. Given the proper lifestyle factors, the subclass B state, if carried in the genes, will be the dominant mode of expression. It's logical that this pattern is being repeated in the children of the one son who is married.

This family tree is revealing, yet the family members at risk would probably pass through most medical care systems completely unaware of their risks until they actually started to have symptoms.

Nobody except the grandfather has any evidence of heart disease. And his two sons have what would be considered "normal" LDL cholesterol levels. Yet both these sons are at risk for heart disease because their father is subclass B and had a heart attack at age fifty-seven. One son, the runner, has probably reversed a lot of his risk by exercising. Now it's time for his brother to follow his example.

The one daughter isn't out of the woods either. She has to be watched very closely as she goes through menopause. There's an even chance she will eventually convert to a subclass B as well.

But my biggest worry is for the nineteen-year-old daughter of the marathon runner. She's already a subclass B, and the combination of a high Lp(a) she inherited from the mother places her at a risk for early heart disease about ten times greater than her cholesterol levels alone would indicate.

Remember: A family history of premature coronary artery disease makes it five times more likely that you too will develop heart disease at an early age.

The array of risk factors I've just discussed is complex, and you need a systematic approach to them. These are the four principles that guide this approach:

- Individualize the pattern of risk factors as much as possible
- Tailor treatments that are specific to the identified risk factors
- Track responses to each intervention with repeat testing before assuming effectiveness or ineffectiveness of any intervention
- Whenever possible, proceed with lifestyle changes first, then medications

How close you need to come to the ideal reductions in risk will depend upon a number of things: whether you already have coronary artery disease, your family history, and the presence of these other risk factors:

- Smoking
- High blood pressure
- Diabetes (either kind)
- Age of 45 or greater for men
- Age of 55 or greater for women (or woman with premature menopause not taking estrogen therapy)
- Obesity

These considerations are important both in the initial choice of what risk factor to check for and the relative danger of that factor. There's a logical format to follow when deciding which tests for hidden risk factors you should take. And there's a systematic pathway for enabling you to determine the level of a risk factor that is right for your unique set of conditions. Chapters 8 through 11 discuss each of these risk factors, taking you through a pathway such that you can see where you fit in. Then you'll know what tests you need and what the results should be for you.

If You Have Coronary Artery Disease

If you have coronary artery disease, you aren't interested in risk. You must dissect the components of your disease and achieve as closely as possible the ideal values for *every* risk factor. This will usually mean stepping beyond lifestyle modifications (diet and exercise) and moving on to medication. Because you already have advanced atherosclerosis, the stepwise approach I will outline for each risk factor is not appropriate. Instead, you should begin behavioral and pharmacological interventions at the same time.

For example, an LDL subclass A person with high LDL levels of 160 would start on the recommended first line medication at the same time as beginning a diet, exercise, and weight loss program. You don't have time to wait for lifestyle modifications to display their full effects, which can take months or even years.

Unless the coronary artery disease patient has revealing test results in family members that point to the presence of specific risk factors, it is absolutely necessary that every test on our risk profile be analyzed.

If You Have a Family History of Heart Disease

Earlier in this chapter you learned how central your genes are to your susceptibility or resistance to heart disease. If coronary artery disease has been diagnosed in your father or brother before the age of fifty-five or your mother or sister before the age of sixty-five, then you have a positive family history of premature heart disease. This alone puts you into the high-risk category and justifies analysis and treatment of your risk factors.

Testing

The person with a positive family history must assess all of the listed factors, just as in the case of the coronary artery disease patient. The same qualifications about shortcuts also apply. If you can have the afflicted family member or members thoroughly tested, positive results narrow the focus for all of the other family members.

Goals

If you are at high risk by virtue of your genetic heritage, but you don't actually have coronary artery disease, then a balance must be struck between expectations and burdens. By burdens, I mean the need, not to mention cost, of having to take medications that are not necessarily innocuous and many of which, while fairly safe, carry a fairly significant list of annoying side effects. If needed, these medications might be your companions for the rest of your life—a sobering realization for a healthy thirty-year-old.

Lifestyle modifications in a person with a positive family history are of great importance. Most of the inheritable risk factors can be attenuated, if not actually "switched off," by adopting the right habits. Invariably, this means weight loss, proper diet for your genetically determined metabolism, and sufficient exercise.

If changes in behavior can't be made, or if the behavioral changes don't neutralize the risk factors, medication must be considered. This will be an individual decision made with regard to your realistic risk and the anticipated burden of a lifelong medication regime.

Some risk factors have treatments that are less burdensome or just more effective. Other risks are very resistant to therapy or require large doses of troublesome drugs. Since so many of these risks are synergistic, maximizing the treatment of the risk or risks more amenable to change can isolate the more resistant risk from its synergistic pals and, if not disarm it, at least contain its damage.

This table shows how the strategy can work for a number of situations. In all cases, smoking should be eliminated, and high blood pressure, diabetes, and obesity should be controlled.

Commonly Encountered Difficult-to-Treat Problems	Countermeasure
Elevated Lp(a)	reduce fibrinogen levels to < 235
	reduce platelet activity with aspirin
	reduce LDL levels to as far below 100 as possible
	convert to LDL subclass A
	eliminate elevated homocysteine levels
	elevate HDL and HDL2 levels *above* ideal mark
	vitamins E and C
Resistantly elevated LDL cholesterol level (see Chapter 8 for what constitutes an "elevated" LDL level for a particular individual)	raise HDL levels *above* ideal mark and achieve total cholesterol/HDL ratio < 4
	vitamins E and C
	aspirin
	convert to subclass A
	eliminate Lp(a), homocysteine, and fibrinogen risks (if applicable)
Resistantly elevated fibrinogen	raise HDL and HDL2 levels *above* ideal mark
	aspirin
	vitamins E and C
	convert to subclass A
	reduce Lp(a) if elevated
	reduce homocysteine if elevated
	reduce LDL < 100

Low HDL	raise HDL2 levels above ideal
	convert to subclass A
	reduce LDL < 100
	aspirin
	vitamins E and C
	treat fibrinogen and homocysteine if elevated
LDL subclass B	lower LDL cholesterol level < 100
	raise HDL and HDL2 levels above ideal mark
	lower total cholesterol/HDL ratio below 4
	aspirin
	vitamins E and C
	identify and eliminate homocysteine,
	fibrinogen, Lp(a) risk

Total Cholesterol: What It Is and How It Is Measured

Total cholesterol includes the cholesterol content of your LDL particles (low-density lipoproteins), your HDL particles (high-density lipoproteins), your VLDL particles (very-low-density lipoproteins), and your IDL particles (intermediate density lipoproteins). Triglycerides are measured separately when you get a blood test.

There is a mathematical relationship among these factors:

$$TC = LDL \text{ cholesterol} + HDL \text{ cholesterol} + (TG/5).$$

The usual way this determination is made is the total cholesterol and the triglycerides are directly measured from your blood sample. Then the LDLs, the IDLs, and VLDLs are thrown out, and the HDLs remaining in the tube are measured. The assumption is made that IDL and VLDL cholesterol equals the TG level divided by 5. Then, knowing the TG (triglycerides) divided by 5, TC and HDL numbers, the LDL cholesterol level is calculated. This method is accurate when the TGs are less than 400 or so. Above that level, distortions of the various molecules introduce errors, and different procedures must be used to ensure accuracy. Even at the extremes of the cholesterol scale this number conveys little useful information for any individual. About 20 percent of people with coronary artery disease have a cholesterol greater than 240. A person with a cholesterol of 240 falls into a risk category where 80 percent of the people in that category will develop coronary artery disease. Yet some of the people who are virtually immune from heart disease have cholesterols in this range.

As you see, the cholesterol number is a composite. It doesn't describe a specific element in the array of atherosclerosis risk factors. Remember, included in the total cholesterol number is LDL (or "bad") cholesterol; HDL ("good") cholesterol; and the cholesterol contained in the precursors to the LDL particles. Each of these entities have completely different roles in atherosclerosis, and a "total cholesterol" number really doesn't tell you anything about their proportions in your blood.

For instance, there will be a few lucky people in the 80 percent risk category whose elevated total cholesterol is the result of an extremely elevated HDL level. These people (provided they lack other risk factors) are nearly immune to heart disease.

For example, take these two men, both with the same total cholesterol:

John		David	
Total cholesterol = 198		*Total cholesterol = 198*	
Triglycerides	140	Triglycerides	140
HDL	70	HDL	35
LDL	100	LDL	135
TC/HDL	2.8	TC/HDL	5.6

HDL comprises a substantial part of John's total cholesterol with a very low LDL. He is in all likelihood an LDL subclass A person (you'll read more about LDL subclasses in the next chapter) with very high levels of HDL2s, and carries a tiny risk for heart disease.

David, with the same total cholesterol number and the same midrange triglyceride level, hides a much different story. His HDLs are in the danger range while his LDL level is just barely acceptable. He is at high risk for heart disease.

One of the more refined population risk markers is the ratio of total cholesterol to HDL—the last line in our example above. It very reliably tells you which risk subgroup you are in, distinguishing the problem profile from the more probably benign profile. Ratios greater than 4 are a warning flag.

Obtaining Your Basic Coronary Artery Disease Risk Profile

Everyone should have the following tests performed by the age of twenty—initial lipid screen: total cholesterol, LDL, HDL, triglyceride, LDL subclass.

Most people can rattle off their Social Security numbers, the 800 number to their stockbroker, and a few key nine- or ten-digit account numbers without hesitation. But ask them for the numbers that more than any others will predict the length and quality of their lives, and you typically hear, "Oh yeah, uh, something around 200. They said everything was normal."

In fact, there is no such thing as a "normal" cholesterol, or a "normal" lipid profile. That's why from the beginning, the first time you even have your blood tested for "cholesterol factors" or a "coronary risk screen," as it's often called, you need a *complete* set of tests performed.

You begin the analysis of your individual profile by reviewing your LDL status, and you must know your LDL subclass to understand it. After LDL, you will then proceed to triglycerides and HDL. In the assessment of each, you will learn where you stand versus the general population, what tests are needed to further define your risk, and what you must do about that risk once you know it. Finally, you will learn how to integrate interventions that have overlapping effects.

There are three general categories of people who require three different levels of aggressiveness in both risk factor evaluation and treatment:

1. The person with no family history of premature coronary heart disease appearing in a sibling or parent.

2. The person *with* such a family history.

3. The person with known coronary artery disease.

The first two groups should start with lifestyle changes, then, if a determined effort fails to have the desired results, add medications later. People in the third group need to make lifestyle changes and take medicine simultaneously. In a sense, the person with coronary artery disease has lost the first battle—but not the war. With aggressive, full-range, and repeated testing, aggressive treatments of each identified risk, with medications that are specific to those risk factors, and the maximization of those treatments as far as the constraints of any individual's tolerance permits, we can now confidently contain and even reverse coronary artery disease in a significant percentage of those who have it.

8

Step Three:
Find Out Your LDL
Level and LDL Subclass

The central risk for heart disease is something you may never have heard of before you picked up this book: the LDL particle. Your risk will be determined by how much cholesterol all of these particles contain (your LDL cholesterol level) and the character of the particles themselves (your LDL subclass).

Your LDL subclass—you can be either A or B—is determined by the distribution of the various sizes and densities of LDL particles in your blood. The more small, dense LDL particles you have, the greater your risk.

Here are the average LDL levels in the American population (values in milligrams per deciliter):

	Male	Female
Average	136	120
Highest 10%	184	168
Lowest 10%	93	82

The LDL cholesterol level indicates the amount of cholesterol contained in all of the LDL particles. Your risk varies according to both the total amount of cholesterol contained in all of your LDL particles and the distribution and size of the different families of LDL particles. The character of these particles also determines what kinds of interventions will be effective in reducing your risk—different kinds of particles respond differently to behavior and medication interventions. So you need to know both your total LDL cholesterol number and your LDL subclass.

73

Determining LDL Subclass

The test available to consumers to distinguish the different types of LDL particles is the LDL gradient gel electrophoresis or LDL-GGE for short. This test samples your LDL cholesterol, using a chemical gel. Different-size LDL particles are separated out by the graded density of the gel. The result reveals a distribution of different-size particles in order of size. It is this distribution of different kinds of particles that determines your LDL subclass.

This test separates the LDL cholesterol content into seven kinds of particles ranging in size from 220 angstroms for the smallest up to 264 angstroms or greater for the largest. The particles called 3A and 3B are the most harmful. If your LDL-GGE determines a peak particle size of greater than 263 angstroms and your LDL3 amount is less than 15 percent of the total, you fall into LDL Subclass A. If your test yields a particle size smaller than 257 angstroms and your LDL3s constitute more than 20 percent of the total, you are in LDL Subclass B.

Many things can affect the distribution of your LDL particle types, and the distribution can change over time in the same person. This happens especially in women around menopause, with people on diet, weight-loss, or exercise programs, or in people who are taking cholesterol-lowering medications.

The Subclass A Population

Subclass A is not benign—half the people who get heart attacks are in this subclass—but risk reduction is often simpler. If you're subclass A, you most accurately conform to the traditional cholesterol-risk model. Your risk can be roughly determined using the American College of Cardiology risk-assessment questionnaire in chapter 5. Your LDL level should be at or below about 130 mg/dl if you have none of the risk factors listed below. If this is so, your LDL situation is good.

Risk Factors

- Smoking
- High blood pressure
- Diabetes (either kind)

- Age of 45 or greater for men
- Age of 55 or greater for women (or women with premature menopause not taking estrogen therapy).
- Obesity
- Sedentary lifestyle

Those with an LDL greater than 130 are at higher risk. Subclass A LDLs from 130 to 159 have an intermediate risk, and LDL levels 160 or greater have a very high risk—at least 100 percent greater than the people below 130. In such people there is so much LDL cholesterol in the arteries that the chances of significant accumulations in the arterial wall are very great.

At the intermediate level of the spectrum, LDL cholesterol of 130 to 159, any of the risk factors listed above amplify the LDL particle's ability to penetrate and accumulate and will move you into a high-risk category. Placing yourself into the right category with respect to your LDL level and life situation is crucial in determining where you need to go from here.

A subclass A person who has an LDL level equal to or greater than 160 or who has an LDL level 130 to 159 plus other risk factors has at least a 100 percent increased risk for developing coronary artery disease. For people in this group who are overweight, achieving weight loss and an exercise level that consumes 2,000 calories or more a week (see chapter 14) is as serious a medical intervention as taking a prescription drug. Many people will never need to take medicines if they can fulfill these goals.

Changing your diet, on the other hand, is a much more problematic issue. You'll find out more about this in chapter 12. Suffice it to say for now that low-fat diets aren't good for everyone. About one-fourth of the general population will actually increase their risk by going on the almost universally advocated low-fat diet. And for such people, the lower the fat, the worse the effects!

Your gender has a great impact on how diet can affect your risk factors. For men, it's not at all certain that you will drop LDL cholesterol levels when adopting a low-fat diet. A great help in predicting which subclass As will respond and which won't is the Apoprotein E isoform test we've mentioned. We'll deal with this test in more detail in chapter 12. Suffice it to say for now that the Apoprotein E test can predict which subclass A person will achieve lower cholesterol in response to a low-fat diet. Moreover, scientific proof that you *will* improve with a particular diet is a great incentive for sticking to it.

The results of this test show that about 25 percent of people will see a substantial reduction (as much as 20 to 25 percent) in LDL level in response to a low-fat diet. But most, the test shows, will respond very little or not at all.

About 15 percent of the population is lucky: They actually *need* fat in their diets. When you place these people on a low-fat diet, triglycerides go up and LDL cholesterol doesn't change. And, even more important, their protective HDL levels can fall— I know, I'm one of them. On a 25 percent fat diet, my LDL cholesterol level rose while my HDLs fell! The tip-off that this is happening might be a large percentage rise in triglycerides.

The Apoprotein E test also reveals a very small number of people who, when placed on a low-fat, high-carbohydrate diet, will see their triglyceride levels shoot up astronomically, into the hundreds or even thousands, increasing just as impressively as their risk for heart disease. Such people will increase their risk for heart disease by adopting a low-fat, high-carbohydrate diet. Fortunately, they are a tiny percentage of the population.

The Apoprotein E test result for most men will place them in the group whose response to the low-fat diet will be unpredictable—at best about half the LDL cholesterol reduction of those whose test predicts the optimal response. For this large group, trial and error is the only approach. Unfortunately, the Apoprotein E test information has yet to be proven useful in predicting how responsive subclass A women are to changes in diet. There is, however, a reason for women to take it.

Apoprotein E represents an independent risk factor for heart disease apart from its ability to predict responses to diet changes. This is true for both sexes. The results of the test can distinguish a group of subclass A men and women who have about a 30 percent increased risk over people with similar LDL cholesterol levels. This distinction adds a new risk factor to a woman's profile, making any risk-lowering intervention all the more important.

Frozen Yogurt and Fat-Free Cake

As you will more and more appreciate, your LDL subclass is more than a type of cholesterol particle. It describes an entire metabolic state of your body. Apart from any Apoprotein E effects, your subclass also describes how fats and sugars are metabolized. Subclass A people on low-fat diets preferentially reduce their large, buoyant LDL A particles, which swing the distribution of their particles toward the small, dense B variety. In studies where subclass A men were put on such diets, as much as 44 percent of the subclass A men shifted this distribution so severely that they actually converted into LDL subclass Bs. Rather than reducing the total number of LDL *particles,* which is the desired result, LDL subclass A particles become denuded of cholesterol while more dense, triglyceride-rich, and cholesterol-poor B particles become more plentiful. Although the LDL cholesterol level may have fallen, risk has not decreased because the diet change has resulted in more of the malignant variety of LDL particles. A clue that an adverse result may be occurring is a substantial rise, 40 to 60 percent, in your original triglyceride level.

In the United States, a low-fat, high-carbohydrate diet usually means eating more commercially processed "low-fat" foods. These foods have high sugar content as opposed to crude, complex carbohydrates. This shift in nutrient balance causes elevations of triglycerides and the consequent deleterious changes of both LDL and HDL particles. This can increase your risk, especially if the shift in distribution is not accompanied by a large reduction in LDL cholesterol per se. Too much fat-free cake and low-fat frozen yogurt can be disastrous.

Medications for Subclass A

Subclass A people specifically respond to certain types of cholesterol-lowering drugs—the "statins": lovastatin, fluvastatin, simvastatin, pravastatin, and atrovastatin. Statins reduce total LDL cholesterol level, and they are effective in reducing the large subclass A particles. But they do not reliably reduce the small, dense, subclass B LDL particles, and they do not alter the distribution profile of the LDL particles. If you are subclass A and just need a reduction in total LDL level, this is good news for you. Your subclass B particles are too few to be the main problem. These subtleties concerning the specific activities of the statins are not always understood even by doctors who prescribe them.

It has been estimated that elevated LDL cholesterol in the subclass A group is the major significant contributor to coronary artery disease in only about 30 percent to 40 percent of the population at risk because of elevated cholesterol. Yet statin drugs are dispensed fairly indiscriminately to people with coronary artery disease. In fact, it is becoming a standard of practice to prescribe a statin for any patient suffering a heart attack who has an LDL above 100. While this is certainly good for the subclass A person, this is not optimal treatment for subclass Bs.

The other drugs that reduce total LDL very effectively are the bile acid binding resins, cholestyramine and colestipol. These two classes of drugs add to the effect of the statins in reducing the A particles, and are also active against the B particles in the distribution. Reduction of either one will result in a fall in the total LDL level, and this is the goal for the subclass A person. These drugs can reduce LDL cholesterol levels to half of original values.

A secondary drug for lowering LDL levels in this group of people is niacin. Niacin primarily lowers small, dense LDL particles, but it is not recommended as primary therapy for the subclass A person. It's an adjunctive treatment to statins or resins for resistantly elevated LDL cholesterol levels.

How low can you go? Don't worry about having an LDL level that is too low. A person needs an LDL level of about *50* in order to maintain normal cellular metabolism, and it is rare for anyone to get to this level even with drugs. For older people, or for those with more risk factors, the lower the LDL the better.

LDL Cholesterol Goals—Subclass A

No risk factors: 130

No risk factors but positive family history or no family history but any other risk factors: Below 130, as close to 100 as possible, especially if multiple risks or diabetes

Family history and risk factors: well below 100

Coronary Artery Disease: well below 100

Most of the North American population have LDL subclass A. If you are married and your spouse is also subclass A, then you can expect this trait to be passed on to your children. Since the genes producing the LDL subclass traits can be turned on and off by so many environmental factors, there are many people who will test positive for subclass A who aren't genetically subclass A at all. They are LDL subclass A because of diet, exercise, and other life conditions (including, for example, being a woman of child-bearing age).

There are many conditions that can cause changes in LDL subclass pattern, and many of them aren't usually thought of as being connected to the risk of heart disease. Your LDL level and your LDL subclass should be checked if you experience any of these changes in your life:

- Change in blood triglyceride level
- Change in diet composition
- Change in total calories in diet
- Change in exercise level
- Change in weight
- Menopause
- Diabetes
- Kidney disease
- Thyroid disease
- Liver disease
- New medications

Subclass A with a Positive Family History

The entire outlook changes if a person has a close family member with premature heart disease. Almost 80 percent of people whose heart disease appears before sixty have an identifiable genetic abnormality that promotes atherosclerosis, and the typical victim of premature heart disease will have *three* genetic risk factors. For these people, reducing the level of LDL cholesterol is not enough—lifestyle modifications and drug therapies targeted at LDL cholesterol reduction may not have an impact on these other hidden genetic abnormalities. Testing for the following factors is necessary:

- Lp(a)
- Homocysteine
- Apoprotein E isoform

- Fibrinogen
- Fasting and two-hour postmeal blood sugar as a screen for hidden diabetes

Subclass A Doesn't Mean You're Out of the Woods

Although the subclass B LDL is much more aggressive in advancing atherosclerotic lesions, about half the people with coronary artery disease are subclass A. If you are an LDL subclass A who develops coronary artery disease despite low LDL cholesterol levels, chances are there are more than one of the non-LDL-related risk factors lurking in your profile. These can be attacked—if you identify them.

Finally, after analyzing all of the other risk factors, there will be a segment of the subclass A population that will have a clean bill of health yet still develop coronary artery disease. There are some subclass A people whose large, buoyant A particles are as susceptible to oxidation as the subclass B particles. As such, they generate atherosclerosis just as aggressively. This is most probably also a genetic trait. There are research procedures that can identify these people, but the tests are not now commercially available.

So the LDL subclass A state can represent the best *and* worst of the heart disease population. It includes those for whom risk may be so low or so controllable that heart disease is a remote possibility, and those who will develop aggressive disease against which at present we have no weapons.

The Subclass B Population

LDL subclass B state is believed to be the product of multiple genes located on at least four different chromosomes. Having LDL subclass B is sometimes called the atherogenic lipoprotein profile, or ALP for short. The subclass B state is more a metabolic syndrome than a single entity, and the small, dense LDL particles that characterize it are as much markers of an atherosclerosis-producing condition as they are active culprits. Subclass B is a condition that mediates the relationships between food digestion, insulin, cholesterol, and triglyceride metabolism, and the chemical structures of all the lipid particles. It is also intimately linked to adult-onset diabetes. In addition, the combination of diabetes with high blood pressure and elevated LDL cholesterol—cardiovascular dysmetabolic syndrome or CDS—seems to be associated with the lipid abnormalities peculiar to subclass B.

As many as half of the men and women with coronary heart disease are LDL subclass B. This is way out of proportion to its presence in the general population. For the same level of LDL cholesterol, the untreated subclass B person has a 300 percent greater risk for developing coronary artery disease than a subclass A counterpart. But with the correct interventions, atherosclerotic lesions "melt" better for LDL subclass B than for subclass A. In fact, you can in many cases halt the process of atherosclerosis and even reverse it.

In the general population, 30 to 35 percent of men and 10 to 12 percent of premenopausal women have the subclass B trait. This percentage doubles for postmenopausal women. In targeting this particle, it is as important to change its behavior as it is to reduce the amount of cholesterol it carries. In other words, the quantity of LDL cholesterol is only part of the story. You have to convert the LDL particle distribution from subclass B to subclass A.

Who Might Have LDL Subclass B?

The LDL subclass B condition is frequently found in people with total LDL cholesterols below 130, the level at which the subclass A person with no other risk factors is considered safe. People with total LDL levels as low as 75 or 80 have been found to still have the subclass B trait; so don't assume a low LDL level means subclass A status.

It is true, however, that people with elevated cholesterol, especially people in the extremely high risk group characterized by LDL cholesterol greater than 160 and total cholesterol over 240, will have a disproportionate clustering of other risk factors, one of which will often be the subclass B state. The combination of HDLs in the low or below average range and triglycerides in the above average range is the classic laboratory warning flag for an underlying LDL subclass B state. For men, this means HDL levels below 40 and triglyceride levels above 125. For women, these numbers are 55 and 90 respectively. These are rough criteria that will include many subclass As and miss many subclass B people. However, the combination has proven to be very useful as a "first pass" indicator that a high risk state may be hiding behind normal lab values.

It has recently been discovered that triglyceride level after a test meal is a fairly sensitive indication of the subclass B state. Much more so than a fasting TG level, this postmeal rise in TGs reveals the body's inability to clear TG fats from the bloodstream after they are absorbed from the intestines.

There are two major groups for whom repeated LDL subclass testing is important throughout life: women after menopause and people who develop adult onset diabetes, otherwise known as non-insulin-dependent diabetes.

About half the women who harbor the genes for the subclass B state have effectively shut those genes off because of their premenopausal hormone balances. This can change when taking oral contraceptives or after menopause, so women should recheck their status at these times. Its presence is a very powerful argument for postmenopausal hormone therapy.

People who develop diabetes later in life also have a greater risk for being subclass B. About half of non-insulin-dependent diabetics will be positive. This represents an extreme risk for coronary artery disease because the metabolic disturbances of the two conditions, and the atherosclerosis-promoting mechanisms they produce, are intimately linked and amplify each other geometrically. The LDL subclass B diabetic is at very high risk for developing coronary artery disease, and particularly if he has high blood pressure.

Obesity is another warning flag that you may have the subclass B state, and it doesn't take much excess fat to activate the subclass B genes. From the body mass index table on page 168, you can see the appropriate weight for your height. The accepted range of weights for an individual's height is actually quite broad, and can hide a serious excess of fat. For more details about this, see Chapter 13.

While anyone who is overweight has an increased risk for developing coronary artery disease, the distribution of the excess fat on the body is another factor to consider. People with what is known as central obesity—those who carry their weight above the belt and along the flanks (a potbelly and love handles)—have a different hormonal mix than those who gain weight in the legs, arms, and buttocks. This hormonal mix affects the production of LDL particles, so having a potbelly is another indicator of the subclass B state. It is also common to find that the person who is overweight around the midriff also has at least the chemical predisposition for diabetes as well as the subclass B.

Finally, medications can also have a negative impact. In fact, some of the most common and effective medications used for the treatment of heart disease can adversely affect the LDL situation. Beta-blockers and thiazide diuretics, both used to treat coronary artery disease, can adversely shift lipid balances. If you have started such medications, you should recheck your "standard" lipid profile and LDL subclass status after about six weeks. An adverse influence of the diuretic may be reason to change to another class of diuretics. Beta-blockers, on the other hand, are powerful, first-line armaments against the symptoms of coronary artery disease. It's rarely justifiable to discontinue them because of a shift in LDL distribution or an increase in LDL level. Rather, you may need to more intensely treat the LDL situation itself.

Managing Subclass B

The approach to reducing coronary artery disease risk in LDL subclass B people is quite different from subclass A. The first step is qualitative: You have to change the nature of the LDL particles from the small dense B particle to the large A particle. This is the first step, regardless of LDL cholesterol level per se, because its success will determine how aggressive the second stage of risk reduction needs to be. If you convert to subclass A, then you can be managed by subclass A criteria.

The steps to take in treating those with subclass B are:

1. Convert it to subclass A.
2. Assess risk according to LDL cholesterol level.
3. Proceed as in subclass A.

The subclass B situation can often be completely taken care of by exercise and weight loss. I know I've said horrible things about these subclass B particles, but they're as malleable as they are malignant.

How do you change B to A? Part of the answer to this is a familiar story: diet, weight loss, and exercise.

Diet

Generally, the subclass B person has a better response to a low-fat diet than does the subclass A person. On a diet that is less than 30 percent fat, a subclass B will significantly reduce his or her *total* LDL cholesterol level but will not normally convert from a B to an A subclass. The level of LDL cholesterol reduction one can expect is extremely variable but can reach as high as 20 percent.

Weight Loss

Dietary changes that result in a significant weight loss may just do the trick. Not only will you lower your LDL cholesterol level, but you also may convert from subclass B to A. So attaining normal weight is a crucial first step in dealing with the subclass B state. But in many cases, diet change and weight loss won't have the desired impact, so what else can you do?

Exercise

As with many other components of the atherosclerosis process, exercise can have a dramatic impact on one's LDL subclass status, and this effect seems dose related—the more you exercise, the better the chance of changing your subclass status. It is also magnified by an associated *fat* weight loss. But losing fat weight, gaining muscle mass, total weight status, and exercise are all factors that are extremely complex and intertwined, making it very difficult to attribute a particular kind of change in your risk profile to a particular intervention.

A proper weight loss diet—losing about two pounds a week— will result in fat reduction. That fat weight loss may be masked by an increase in muscle mass from the exercise. The net result, however, will be a reduction in one's LDL cholesterol and very possibly a shift in LDL subclass. Your scale may not notice anything, but your heart will.

The more calories per week you use up when exercising the more likely this is to happen. Subclass Bs should strive for a minimum of 2,000 calories of exercise a week. Moreover, this amount of exercise should be performed at an intensity level that is greater than 400 calories per hour. That's equal to about a 4 mph run. (See chapter 14 for the details on exercise.) After about six to eight weeks of diet, weight loss, and exercise, your blood tests should be rechecked to see if further interventions will be needed. If the blood tests show that you need more, it's time for medication.

Medication for Subclass B

The required medications are niacin, the fibric acid derivatives, and the bile acid binding resins. Niacin is usually the first line of attack. It can be expected both to change the subclass B pattern to an A pattern and reduce the total LDL level—a nice response, especially when LDL is elevated.

If niacin therapy has reversed the subclass B to A but the total LDL level is still too high, a statin can be added for the final step of reducing LDL to your goal level. That level is as close to 100 as possible for a person with other risk factors. Someone without risk factors should be below 130 (see page 78).

As with any of these drug combinations, adding a second drug usually allows you to take less of each for the same effect. This is particularly important if either drug is producing side effects. The smaller the dose you can get away with, the less chance for side effects. That's especially true of niacin, and with niacin there is a catch. The doses of niacin required are gigantic when compared to what's in even the most powerful multivitamin. For niacin to act on your risk factors, it must be taken in doses of 1 gram or more. And at these levels, almost everyone using standard niacin tablets will initially experience unpleasant side effects unless the dose is gradually built up over many weeks or even months and the right formulation is used. That's why if you and your doctor are contemplating using niacin you should read chapter 15 carefully, since there is a more gentle niacin formulation available.

The bile acid binding resins are effective in treating both LDL types but are usually even more effective for the subclass B patient. They're not the first choice, though, because with some subclass B patients, they will reduce LDL levels but increase other undesirable lipid levels like triglycerides. So these drugs may not be a good single therapy for subclass B.

Fibric acid drugs, on the other hand, can be used as both single, first-line therapy or, more commonly, in combination with either niacin or a statin. These drugs are very active against the small dense LDL particles, reliably causing conversion to the subclass A pattern. This is particularly true if your triglycerides are above 200. In that case, this may be the only drug needed.

Fibric acid drugs won't lower the total LDL levels the way niacin does. If they are to be used as single agents, the perfect patient would be one with high triglycerides who needs to have his LDL converted from subclass B to A but who does not need a reduction in total LDL levels.

So the subclass B person commonly requires a combination of two or three drugs, whereas the subclass A person often gets away with one drug, a statin. The combination drug regimens usually are:

niacin: statin

niacin: fibric acid

niacin: resin

fibric acid: statin

niacin: fibric acid: statin

niacin: fibric acid: resin

Don't be discouraged by the panoply of pills and powders you might find yourself taking. Though the subclass A person with just a high LDL cholesterol level usually has an easier therapeutic time of it, if such a person does go on to get coronary artery disease despite this aggressive prevention and low relative risk, that person becomes very difficult to treat.

On the other hand, the subclass B person undertaking aggressive preventative steps is extremely sensitive to treatment. Studies have shown that although untreated atherosclerosis proceeds twice as fast in subclass Bs as in subclass As, subclass Bs are much more likely to see cholesterol plaque melt away with treatment. And if the subclass B person does develop symptomatic coronary artery disease, it is much easier to prevent it from progressing.

The subclass B person should undertake whatever interventions are necessary for conversion to subclass A, then wait and see. If you convert to subclass A and never develop heart disease, or if your already present disease stabilizes or regresses and LDL levels are OK, there is no need to worry about any remaining harmful LDL subclass B particles. But if the disease continues to progress, intensified treatment may be necessary. Sometimes therapy for those who are subclass B will obliterate the overtly lethal qualities from the LDL-GGE results, converting the person to a subclass A, or at least an intermediate pattern. But such therapy might still leave some disturbing forms of LDL particles as minor peaks in the 3- or 4-particle range of the LDL-GGE test. If no other risk factor has been overlooked, the object of further treatment will be to minimize the number of harmful LDL particles by intensifying the treatment against the B particles. Remember, every person has the entire spectrum of LDL particles. Treatment shifts the distribution of particles and reduces their total number but doesn't eliminate any kind of particle completely.

How to Guess Your Subclass without Taking the Blood Test

Triglyceride Levels

It may not be easy or convenient to get the special test that tells for sure which LDL subclass you belong to. But there may be enough information in your standard lipid profile to make a good guess which subclass you are in. The key element in making this guess is your triglyceride level. When you eat fat, it is digested by the enzymes in the cavities of your stomach and intestine. This digestion liberates millions of molecules called triglycerides, which are then absorbed into the bloodstream, where they are herded into large clumps called chylomicrons. In some people these clumps can be so large that you can see them with the naked eye floating in a blood sample. In the circulation, the clumped triglycerides are very rapidly broken down into their basic fat molecules, the fatty acids. These are then absorbed as "food" by various cells in the body.

The enzyme that disperses this triglyceride into the morsels of fat used as food by the body's cells is LPL, lipoprotein lipase (no relation to LDL). This is the key enzyme in moving triglycerides from the bloodstream into the hungry cells, which will literally vaporize those fatty acids into heat and the gases you ultimately exhale from your lungs—a useful end that all fats should, but unfortunately do not, experience.

LPL lines the blood vessels, so triglycerides, as long as they are circulating in the blood, can't hide from it. How effective your LPL is in getting rid of triglycerides depends on the amount of LPL you have, the amount of fat you're presenting to it, and the target cells' appetite for that fat.

Any imbalance in this triangle can result in triglycerides accumulating in the bloodstream. Even if you eat no fat at all, your liver still produces triglycerides, and all it needs to do so is enough carbohydrates. Just as fat is broken down into triglycerides, carbohydrates are broken down into sugar by your digestive tract and then pumped into the circulation. Once there, the sugar's fate is determined by a different triangular balance of factors.

The amount of sugar must be balanced against the appetite of the cells that use the sugar as food. Insulin facilitates entry of sugar into a cell. When there's more sugar than the cells want, or the amount of sugar presented to the circulation is too much for the insulin to handle, it goes back to the liver, which transforms it into triglyceride for eventual storage as fat. That's why if you eat too much bread or pasta, you become just as fat, just as quickly, as if you ate too many hamburgers and fries.

Moving things around the body requires some kind of molecular transport system. In the case of fats, the molecular transports are the LDL particle, the chylomicrons we've already mentioned, and certain other particles related to the LDL particle, among them the VLDLs (very low density lipoprotein), and IDLs (intermediate-density lipoproteins).

The liver takes the excess triglycerides we've eaten, the triglycerides it has manufactured from the excess carbohydrates we've eaten and the relatively small amount of cholesterol it has manufactured for the cells that need it and bundles them into a VLDL particle that it ejects into the circulation. Then a complex system of protein markers steers the VLDL particles to the organs waiting to digest the fats they contain.

Now the LPL enzymes go into action. They ambush these VLDL particles as they go by and pick off triglyceride molecules. The effect is to slenderize the VLDL particle into a new creature, the IDL—the intermediate-density lipoprotein—which is not only smaller than the VLDL but also now contains a much higher percentage of cholesterol mixed with the remaining triglycerides.

These IDLs are largely cleared by the liver, but the predation by LPL on those remaining IDLs produces the final transformation of this particle into the troublesome LDL, which is comprised mainly of the remaining cholesterol, the triglyceride not stolen by LPL, and the Apoprotein B protein marker.

The more triglyceride there is available for incorporation into the VLDL molecule, the harder it will be for all of those scavengers and predators to denude this transport particle of its triglyceride. Hence the more triglyceride remaining, the more poisonous the final LDL personality.

The amount of triglyceride left in the LDL particle partly determines its size, its density, and its chemical personality. The interaction of all these metabolic factors determines how much triglyceride is left in the LDL particle and, therefore, whether you're a subclass A or a subclass B.

Still, inferring LDL subclass from triglyceride level is perilous, and made more so by the variations in triglyceride levels in blood samples from the same person at different times. Triglyceride levels vary radically from one hour to the next, depending on when, what, and how much you've eaten. It's extremely important to test triglycerides early in the morning after an overnight fast, preferably twelve to sixteen hours long. That's when your triglyceride level will reflect the baseline character of your metabolism. If you do it this way, there might be some utility in substituting a triglyceride level for an LDL subclass determination—at least for some people.

If your triglycerides are very low—below 75—you are almost surely subclass A; if they are above 180, you are more likely to be subclass B. In the middle ranges, however, only the LDL subclass blood test will tell you for sure. Since 80 percent of men's triglycerides fall in the 66 to 265 range and 80 percent of women's in the 55 to 182 range, most people will still have to have the LDL subclass test in order to determine their subclass. Thus using triglyceride levels to reliably substitute for the LDL subclass test will only be valid for less than one person out of ten. But even with all this uncertainty, triglyceride levels are still very useful as a warning sign that you may have an undetected subclass B state.

A more accurate though more involved way to use triglyceride levels is to test the level six hours after a test meal. Failure to efficiently clear the blood of these fats is very suggestive of subclass B state. This "clearance failure" may easily hide beneath unremarkable fasting TG levels.

The importance of lifestyle changes, weight loss, exercise, and diet now fall into place. If you exercise, you increase the muscle cells' appetite for both sugar and triglycerides, clearing both commodities more rapidly from the bloodstream. By changing your diet, you put less of these substances into the bloodstream to begin with. The ultimate result is less triglyceride available to your liver, which means less triglyceride in the VLDL particle, which means, eventually, less triglyceride in the LDL particle. So when you evaluate your triglyceride level, don't just look at the absolute level. Think about those triangles. If you're working very hard to influence those relationships and you come up only "normal," there's a good chance subclass B is lurking despite a low normal triglyceride test report.

Finally, remember that this is a genetic disorder. Because of their genetic makeup, there are people who, no matter how drastically they affect the balances of our two triangles in favor of low triglycerides, will still produce a subclass B particle distribution, while there are others who need only a modification of diet or exercise level to shift into a subclass A pattern.

Inferring LDL Subclass from HDL Levels

HDL level, like triglyceride level, can also suggest what subclass you're in, even if you don't get the subclass blood test. One of the most consistent antagonisms in human metabolism is the relationship between triglyceride and HDL levels. As the former rises, the latter falls, and vice versa. So low HDL levels also suggest subclass B status. The relationship can be very subtle, varying only by a few percentage points each way, especially in people whose lipid screen values are in all respects well within the "normal" ranges.

About 30 percent of subclass A people will have HDL values below 40 mg/dl, which is a low "normal" number, and about 30 percent of subclass B people will have an HDL above 40 mg/dl. This is the point where the two sets of relationships cross. As a rule of thumb, an HDL below 40 suggests subclass B, while one above 40 suggests subclass A. Virtually all LDL subclass B people will have an HDL less than 70, but so will most subclass As. Since the percentage of subclass B people above an HDL level of 50 is very small, being over 50 strongly suggests subclass A.

Almost 30 percent of subclass Bs will have an HDL above 40 and, conversely, about 30 percent of subclass As will have an HDL below 40. Thus, for most people, HDL levels, like triglycerides, only give a probable indication of LDL subclass.

Inferring Subclass B from Apoprotein B Levels

The Apoprotein B test quantifies the actual number of LDL particles you have rather than the amount of cholesterol they contain (the LDL cholesterol level), or the distribution of the particles' sizes and densities (the LDL subclass). A subclass B person will have more particles than a subclass A person for the same amount of LDL cholesterol. If the Apoprotein B level divided by the LDL cholesterol level is greater than 1.1, the chances are very good that you are an LDL subclass B.

9

Step Four:
Find Out Your HDL
(Good Cholesterol) Profile

Like LDL, HDL is a particle floating in your bloodstream. It is composed of cholesterol, triglyceride, and protein "steering" molecules called Apoprotein A-1 and A-II, or Apo A-1, A-II. But unlike the LDL particles, which constitute the greatest single threat to your life, the HDL particles are powerful protectors. They undo just about all the horrible things the LDL particles do.

This protective power of HDL is demonstrated by epidemiological studies. Whereas a one point fall in LDL level yields a 2 percent decrease in one's risk of developing coronary artery disease, the corresponding one point rise in HDL level can—depending on which group of data we use—result in anywhere from a 2.5 to 4 percent decrease in risk.

In a study conducted in a part of Finland that has the highest death rate from coronary artery disease in the world, men who were at the lowest quarter of the HDL scale were more than three times as likely to develop coronary artery disease as the men at the upper quarter of the scale. Similar numbers come out of the Framingham Study.

The Physicians' Health Study also produced interesting results. Though heart attack victims were found to have the same cholesterol levels as the control population, people developing heart attacks were distinguishable by their low HDL levels. Yet most therapy for heart disease prevention is directed at lowering LDL—which clearly does not help everyone—rather than raising HDL.

Differences Between Bad and Good Cholesterol

LDL	HDL
Easily oxidized, intensifying most other mechanisms	Prevents oxidation of LDL
Infiltrates endothelial cells of arterial wall	Diminishes affinity of LDL particle to stick to endothelial cells
Forms accumulations of particles beneath endothelial cell lining	Inhibits LDL aggregation (clumping) and draws cholesterol away from artery wall
Stimulates scavenger cell ingestion of cholesterol	Inhibits scavenger cells' LDL ingestion
Causes overaccumulation of cholesterol in bodies of scavenger cells	Inhibits scavenger cell ingestion
Transforms scavenger cells to foam cells, the beginning of atherosclerosis	Inhibits scavenger cell transformation
Perpetual accumulation in growing plaque	Active reuptake of cholesterol from formed plaque
Stimulates platelets to attach to plaque and accumulate	Inhibits platelet activity
Stimulates alterations of chemical milieu around plaque	Stabilize chemical milieu around plaque
Stimulates clot formation at plaque site	Inhibits clot formation and stimulates clots lysis ("melting")
Stimulates plaque rupture and acute coronary events	Stabilizes plaque capsule
Recirculates cholesterol, causing reformation and replenishment of LDL particles	Promotes transport of circulating and peripherally deposited cholesterol for removal by liver
Stimulates local blood vessel constrictors	Inhibits local blood vessel constrictors
Inhibits local blood vessel dilators	Promotes local blood vessel dilation

In assessing your HDL status, which is the third component of the standard lipid screen triumvirate, be aware that your sex has a profound impact on the evaluation of the numbers. Much more so than with LDL, and to a degree similar to triglycerides, your sex places you on one of two very different scales.

HDL Cholesterol (mg/dl)

Men		
Lowest 10%	*Average*	*Highest 10%*
29	40	57

Women		
Lowest 10%	*Average*	*Highest 10%*
38	55	78

Even the National Cholesterol Educational Program is uncertain about the issue of what is a normal or adequate HDL cholesterol level. These guidelines draw the line at 35 mg/dl as an acceptable HDL for men and women. Yet it is clear that there is a sharp acceleration of risk below the 42 mark. In the Finnish study I mentioned, for example, 35 was well into that doomed-to-get-a-heart-attack lowest quarter of the HDL cholesterol range. Moreover, a correspondingly acceptable HDL cholesterol for a woman is about 10 points higher than that for a man.

Here are the ranges:

HDL Levels

Average	Borderline	Low
Male: 40	Male: 30–40	Male: < 30
Female: 50–55	Female: 40–50	Female: < 40
average risk	high risk	extreme risk

HDL levels are fragile. For instance, a diet change, a new medication for some unrelated condition, or a small weight change might not dent an LDL level but may have a surprising effect on HDL level.

What Is an Adequate HDL?

"I'm running three miles a day. Why can't my HDLs get over 45?" This is a common question coming from an athletic middle-aged man or woman. Usually the situation is more complicated.

Influences That Increase HDL

Weight loss, if overweight

Exercise

Normal or high-fat diet (35 to 40% fat)

Estrogens

Alcohol

Antacid medications: Zantac, Tagamet, Pepcid

Influences That Decrease HDL

Weight gain from normal weight

Sedentary lifestyle

High carbohydrate diet less than 30% fat

High polyunsaturated fat diets

Progesterone

Anabolic steroids

Testosterone

Beta-blocker cardiac medications

Age

Smoking

Liver disease

Kidney disease

Thyroid disease

Athletic people may also be on a low-fat, high-carbohydrate diet—a so-called performance diet. And they may have lost weight on their diet and exercise program. So three different forces are at work. The weight loss and exercise cause HDL levels to rise, but the low-fat diet makes them fall. As this is happening, our middle-aged athlete is experiencing the normal decline in HDL attributable to age, and for the woman, her menopausal status may also be coming into play.

As is the case with LDL, the acceptable level of HDL is an individual matter. Though an average level of HDL might be okay for someone with absolutely no risk factors, a value over 50 for men and over 60 for women is much more appropriate for most people. It is important to review the list of positive and negative factors and see what changes you're capable of making.

There is a very ominous statistic buried in the mountain of data generated by the Framingham Study. The average HDL level of men having coronary artery disease was 43. The average HDL level of women having coronary artery disease was 53—almost identical to what's considered normal for the general population. From this same data pool, the HDL values in people with *premature* coronary artery disease are quite different, however. For those who developed coronary artery disease before the age of sixty, the average HDL was 36.

The distributions of HDL values among the people with coronary artery disease and those without have a tremendous overlap, though not nearly as much as for LDL. There is a sharp drop in the number of people suffering from heart disease when HDL levels rise above 50. By that level, we've accounted for more men than women. It's actually the women, with their average value of 53, who account for most of the casualties at the higher levels of the HDL distribution curve. So you should push your HDL level at least 10 points higher than the average for your gender. How can you accomplish this?

Our middle-aged runner could be helped by some easy adaptations. Changing from a diet of less than 30 percent fat to one of 30 to 40 percent fat might be all he needs to reverse the situation. Eating more fish and monounsaturated fats is the best way to do this. While you can't do anything about your age, a woman's falling HDL levels after menopause may be one more factor to weigh when deciding whether to use hormone replacement therapy.

And then there's exercise. Most people who think they exercise adequately—even vigorously—don't do enough to impact HDL levels. We'll go into much more detail in Chapter 14 about how much and how intensely you should exercise to really change your HDL level. For now, realize that the exercise effect is dose dependent. The more you do, the better.

With the exception of age, menopause, and the presence of actual diseases, the list of factors affecting HDL levels is largely a list of behavioral modifications and medications. But of course metabolism and genetic makeup also play a role.

Triglyceride level and LDL subclass status are half of the influences on HDL level. All of the factors appearing on the list will have variable and often unpredictable effects, depending on the state of your metabolism. High triglyceride levels can cause HDLs to fall. This is part of the picture of the subclass B state. Falling triglycerides may signal a rise in HDLs, just as they may signal a conversion from the LDL subclass B to subclass A state.

Because triglycerides, HDLs, and LDLs are all linked, many of the same interventions are effective in optimizing all three. But in some cases the effects are antagonistic: What raises an HDL (like more fat in the diet) level may promote the subclass B state and raise LDL levels. This can be very tricky to manage—even with professional help. Just when we think we've got it all figured out, more convolutions erupt. For example, let's look at diet.

A low-fat, high-carbohydrate diet that is not intended to gain or lose weight may cause a fall in HDL levels. You've learned that the effect of various diets on LDL, however, is highly variable, depending on subclass and, in some cases, on your Apoprotein E test results.

The tables below show how, and how much, different behavioral modifications can affect HDL levels—the more + signs, the more positive the effect. Remember: Impacts are relative. Absolute number changes for any individual can't be predicted.

What Raises HDL Levels?

For a Person on a 35% to 40% Fat Diet	
Exercise	++
Weight Loss	+++
Exercise with weight loss	++++
No exercise or weight loss	Level remains stable

What Raises HDL Levels?

For a Person on a High-Carbohydrate Diet That Is Less than 30% Fat	
Exercise	+
Weight Loss	++
Exercise with weight loss	+++
No exercise or weight loss	Decline in level

Low HDL

Having a persistently low HDL is a serious problem. If after making all the lifestyle adjustments you can, your HDL is still in the unacceptable range, the two most likely possibilities are that you are an LDL subclass B (more likely) or you have a condition called hypoalphalipoproteinemia, or Hypo A for short (less likely). In other words, the problem is in your genes. If this is the case, you need some help in the form of medication. In the case of resistantly low HDL associated with subclass B, the first line medication treatments for subclass B are also potent HDL boosters. Niacin is a powerful HDL stimulant, and fibrates will prove particularly helpful if TGs are above 200.

Low HDL and the Apoprotein A-1 Test

There are some people whose low HDL levels are not accounted for by the LDL subclass B state, high triglycerides, or behavioral or lifestyle factors. There are others who after conversion of their subclass B state still have very low HDLs. These people remain at high risk. In both cases, confirmation of the low HDL is important because the implications can be very serious, and this confirmation requires a different test.

Some people just can't get consistently accurate HDL blood levels drawn. Much of this has to do with the methodology of the standard HDL test. To rule out this possibility, a test called the Apoprotein A-1 test can be used to confirm the low HDL condition. This test actually measures the protein "tag" of the HDL particle rather than the cholesterol part. This results in a more accurate measure of how many HDL particles the person is producing. Though this test is less common, it's much easier to do accurately. Values lower than 90 mg/dl for men and 100 for women are in the lowest 10 percent of the population and correspond to the low HDL levels obtained earlier.

Hypo A is a genetic disorder, and it is very deadly. In the classic Framingham Offspring Study, 40 percent of people who developed heart disease before the age of sixty had this problem either alone or in combination with other factors.

It is believed that Hypo A exists in less than 10 percent of the general population, so it's uncommon but not rare. And it is present in about 20 percent of all coronary artery disease patients. Fifty percent of the children of an affected parent can be affected, so when this condition is discovered, it is absolutely crucial to go up and down the genetic ladder, testing parents and children.

As with most of these genetic disorders, its sensitivity to being turned on and off by other factors varies from person to person. All the factors, both metabolic and behavioral, that cause HDLs to fall can radically amplify this condition. So treatment starts with clearing your lungs of tobacco smoke and your blood of excess triglycerides. Despite this, most true Hypo A-1s won't appreciably improve without medication. They just aren't equipped to manufacture HDL.

That's when niacin should be tried, but unlike all the other situations for which niacin seems like a miracle drug, against the Hypo A-1 gene (or genes) it often finds its match; they don't respond. Postmenopausal women have another option: estrogen therapy.

If there's no response, the best advice medicine has to offer at the present time is to optimize every other metabolic and behavioral risk factor. In short, your goals are identical to the profile results I advised for the person with active coronary artery disease.

The Problem of the "Average" HDL Level

As there are with LDL, there are different kinds of HDL. But their relative significance as atherosclerotic risk factors is not nearly as well understood as it is with the LDL types.

Analogous to the LDL-GGE test, which separates different LDL particles, the HDL-GGE test separates the HDL fraction of the blood into two families of particles, HDL2 and HDL3. Remember that Finnish study where the men with HDL levels below 42 had over a three times increased risk of having a heart attack? Well, when they divided the men by their HDL2 and HDL3 levels, they found that the relative risk of having a heart attack for those men who had the lowest levels of HDL2 was 400 percent, while those with the lowest HDL3s had a 200 percent increased risk. Thus, the HDL2 was twice as protective as the HDL3 and even more protective than the total HDL level itself. HDL2 seemed to be the most important protective factor against coronary artery disease, so much so that a decreased level was more dangerous than elevations of LDL cholesterols, smoking, or high blood pressure.

Still, there is no general agreement about the exact relative significance of these families of HDL. Some studies have shown that HDL3 is more important, and others that total HDL is all that matters.

We can leave the resolution of this issue to the researchers, but there's no debate about the protective value of HDL2. It is sometimes important to make sure that your HDL composition is in a normal balance if the HDL is to do its job effectively. And the situation where this may be crucial is when your total HDLs are in the borderline or low normal range: for men, this means in the range between 30 and 50; for women, between 40 and 60. This range includes a large number of people.

The major task of the HDL particle is to melt atherosclerotic lesions. HDLs float by in the bloodstream, target a cholesterol deposit down in the lining of the artery, and carry it back to the liver for disposal. HDL3s are thin, hungry HDL particles that when they become engorged with cholesterol become HDL2s. It's the HDL2s then that are actually bringing the cholesterol away for disposal. This is called reverse cholesterol transport. It is probably the single most important event occurring in your body ensuring longevity—it is the biological antidote to atherosclerosis.

Normal HDL2 Fractions

Female 45%
Male 25%
For men, more than 25% of your total HDL should be HDL2.
For women, more than 45% of your total HDL should be HDL2.

These relative percentages ensure that at average total HDL values, there are enough HDL2 particles disposing of enough cholesterol to counter the atherosclerotic process. An effectively functioning plaque-melting system has an HDL2 level that is about 25 percent of the total HDL value in men and 45 percent in women. An HDL2 value over these average values indicates that this cholesterol disposal system is beefed up, and an HDL2 percentage of about 45 in men and 65 in women means this system is functioning extremely well.

The problem with "average" HDL cholesterol levels is that if you are accumulating HDL3s and not generating HDL2s, there may not be enough HDL2 particles reabsorbing the cholesterol deposits in your arteries. The absolute number of HDL2 particles is the important thing. If the test shows a high HDL level, there are almost certainly enough HDL2 particles; if it shows a very low level, it is safe to assume that there are not enough HDL2 particles. It's at the average levels that the ratio of HDL2 to HDL3 becomes important. That's when you need to check it.

For example, a man starting an exercise program who starts out with a total HDL cholesterol of 45 but only 10 percent HDL2 is in a dangerous situation. After beating his brains out for six months in four different sports, he checks his HDLs to find they've only risen to 48. This is a very negative incentive for him to continue his new lifestyle. However, if he doesn't check his HDL level through the GGE test, he won't know that his HDL2 distribution has moved to 50 percent! That's a big change for the better and means the exercise is doing exactly what he wants it to do.

On the other hand, this same man's friend who also has an HDL of 45 and HDL2s of 10 percent, starts drinking a glass or two of wine each day while watching television each night. His HDLs increase to 50, but they're almost all HDL3. So while he's bragging to his friend how he accomplished the same reduction in heart disease risk watching television that his friend did by sweating and laboring, the joke's on him. He's not that much better off than when he started.

Most of the same drugs that raise HDL levels also cause favorable swings in HDL distribution, increasing HDL2 more than HDL3. So how far can you take these levels? There's no limit to maximum HDL cholesterol, and there's almost no upper limit to

HDL2 percentage that can be attained. Enough exercise can actually raise the HDL2 percentage to nearly 100. In the case of both HDL and HDL2, the more the better. From the data of that Finnish study, it's been calculated that if everyone's HDL level could be raised to 58 or so, as many as two-thirds of all heart attacks could be prevented.

As you now understand, there is a balance between your HDL particles and all of the other cholesterol particles. This balance is reflected in the relative amount of cholesterol contained in these opposing camps. By dividing your *total* (not just LDL) cholesterol number by your HDL cholesterol number, you derive the total cholesterol/HDL ratio. This is a useful number, because it is a shortcut to tracking your progress in reducing risk.

The effect of interventions should cause this ratio to fall. People without heart disease but without multiple risk factors should have a ratio below 4. People with heart disease or otherwise at high risk must be at or below 3.5. Remember that while this ratio is a useful guide in measuring your progress, it is not a substitute for the risk-factor-focused analysis we've been discussing.

10

Step Five:
Discover Your Lp(a) Level

The Lp(a) is an LDL particle with an extra apoprotein, the Apoprotein A, attached to it. Here are the normal ranges of Lp(a):

	Average	Level of Highest 10% of the Population
Men	3.8 mg/dl	18 mg/dl
Women	4.4 mg/dl	21 mg/dl

Who Should Get the Test

Anyone with any of the following conditions should be tested for Lp(a):

- Coronary artery disease—especially when contemplating coronary bypass surgery or angioplasty.
- Family history of premature coronary artery disease, stroke
- Peripheral vascular disease
- Cerebral vascular disease
- Elevated fibrinogen and homocysteine levels
- Smoking
- Diabetes

What Lp(a) Does

The structure of Apoprotein A is very similar to the structure of another protein circulating in the blood: plasminogen. This protein helps dissolve the blood clots that form around ruptured atherosclerotic plaques. Lp(a), however, with its Apoprotein a attached, can trick the receptors lining the arterial wall responsible for activating plasminogen, thus thwarting the body's response to inappropriate clot formation. In addition, Apoprotein a seems to stimulate the movement of structural cells from the interior of the artery toward the surface to help build up the growing plaque even further. And it is extremely amenable to oxidation, making it a very effective participant in the entire range of activities that go into plaque formation. All of this makes for a very nasty particle that nobody should want to have in any appreciable concentrations.

Genetics and Lp(a)

Elevated Lp(a) is inherited—50 percent of children are likely to have it if a parent does. As with LDL, not all Lp(a)s are alike. Genetic variants of the Apoprotein a gene produce large-, small-, and intermediate-size versions of the protein. African Americans, in whom elevated Lp(a) is more common than in many other populations, may have the intermediate size, which is believed to be less harmful. The large and small sizes are believed to steer Lp(a) into different avenues of mischief.

Unfortunately, the tests to determine genetic variants of Lp(a) are not yet commercially available, so you must approach this issue as if you had all the variants.

Because of its link to the blood-clotting system, Lp(a) has been implicated in causing coronary obstruction in situations that are already prone to enhanced clot formation—in reocclusions of coronary arteries opened by angioplasty and in early failure of coronary artery bypass *vein* grafts, but not grafts made from other *arteries*. For example, in a Japanese study of eighty patients undergoing angioplasty to reopen coronary arteries with high-level blockages by atherosclerotic plaques, 18 risk factors were measured to see which ones were associated with reocclusion of the newly opened arteries. Of all the risk factors recorded, only Lp(a) was correlated with redevelopment of the blockage in the newly opened artery. These results were remarkably similar to an American study of men undergoing angioplasty. Here, too, Lp(a) levels were the only predictors of reocclusion of the coronary artery

High Lp(a) levels have also been associated with increased incidence of atherosclerotic obstructions of other arteries—those supplying the brain and legs, for example.

About one-third of coronary artery disease patients have elevations of Lp(a), which is now considered an independent risk factor for heart disease. There are some studies that show a lack of increased risk in the presence of low LDL levels. However, there may be a synergy between LDL subclass B particles and Lp(a) particles. High LDL levels, especially coupled with high triglyceride levels, act in synergy with Lp(a) to cause cholesterol accumulation in the arterial wall, so Lp(a) is a problem not only late in the disease but also at its earliest stages.

Lp(a) and Risk

An increased risk of about three times has been associated with levels above 25 to 30—about the same as the risk associated with total cholesterol levels in excess of 240 or HDL levels below 35. But the risk of elevated Lp(a) goes up radically in the presence of other risk factors. Lp(a) levels greater than 55 along with total cholesterol to HDL ratios greater than 5.9 carry an astronomical sixteen times greater risk of actually having coronary artery disease. Because of Lp(a)'s tight link to the blood clotting system, people with other coronary artery disease risk factors that also contribute to clotting (such as high fibrinogen levels, high homocysteine levels, or elevated platelet counts) should pay particular attention to their Lp(a) levels.

Treatment

Treatment can be frustrating. It used to be believed that exercise lowered Lp(a) levels, but that's been proven untrue. No diet or other lifestyle changes directly help either. Niacin may be helpful, but it's very hard to build up to sufficient doses without causing unpleasant side effects. While daily niacin doses in the range of 1 to 2 grams are often effective in raising HDLs or converting subclass B, doses of 4 grams or more are often required to substantially lower Lp(a) levels.

Results similar to those with niacin can be obtained with estrogen therapy in postmenopausal women and, most recently, with the estrogenlike anticancer drug tamoxifen. In men, testosterone has been shown to effectively reduce Lp(a) levels.

As with any risk factor, how aggressively one needs to pursue treatment is dependent on the presence of other risks. If Lp(a) is an isolated genetic problem, then the treatment is to eliminate any environmental or lifestyle risks you may have. But if you have a family history of premature coronary artery disease or if you already have heart disease yourself, you should address this problem more directly. Elevated Lp(a), especially in people with heart disease or with a family history of it, or people with other genetic risk factors, can be treated by aggressively reducing other risks. An LDL level of 90 or 100 is good for most people, but in the presence of high Lp(a) resistant to therapy, it may be better to drive the LDL down into the 60s.

Of extreme importance, especially for the person with heart disease, are the other factors that increase blood clotting, homocysteine, and fibrinogen. In the presence of elevated Lp(a), you absolutely must know those levels as well and minimize them if elevated. It's much easier to reduce a homocysteine or fibrinogen level than it is to reduce an Lp(a) level.

11

Step Six:
Understand Your
Blood-Clotting System

There are few moments in medicine as rewarding as the complete reversal of a heart attack. In emergency rooms, cardiac catheterization labs, and cardiac care units all over the world, people who a few years ago would be either doomed or condemned to a lifetime of incapacity because of a heart attack are now being discharged from the hospital as if nothing had happened. This is because we've figured out how to eliminate the blood clot that represents the culmination of the lifelong process of atherosclerosis in the coronary artery. Either by injecting a chemical that immediately dissolves the clot or by piercing it with a catheter that blasts it away, we can reopen the coronary artery channel to allow blood flow to the jeopardized heart muscle.

This dramatic climax is the end of a process that has been progressing for decades, a process intimately connected to one of the normal functions of a healthy body: blood clotting.

There's no more essential aspect of the healing process than the clotting of the blood. No matter what's ripped, clawed, bitten, speared, or crushed, it can't even begin to mend unless the blood spilling through it is stopped. Perhaps even more important than the healing of the damaged tissue is this conservation of the precious blood itself. The body has a mechanism to conserve blood while at the same time not blocking it from flowing to injured sites, because the cells that repair torn tissue and guard its vulnerable borders from invasion from bacteria have to get to the injury via the blood flow to it. The system allows just enough blood flow for repair and nutrition while checking any excess.

In this system, the clotting action is balanced by an anticlotting mechanism. This mechanism is called the fibrinolytic system, and it actually dissolves the clot as fast as it forms. When the system works properly, the clot that forms will be in proportion to the size of the injury that needs it, and the fibrinolytic system will dissolve any excess.

Many experts believe that the actual first moment of the atherosclerotic process has nothing to do with cholesterol at all but with a microscopic injury to the vessel wall, an injury that can be caused by a "natural" factor like high levels of adrenalinelike hormones, or unnatural factors like cigarette smoke. In this conception, the first element of the atherosclerotic process is the attraction of the clotting mechanisms to the injured site of the arterial wall.

Platelets and Clot Formation

Platelets are tiny cells that are attracted to injured tissue of any kind, where they accumulate to stop the flow of blood and then chemically stimulate the clotting cascade to begin. A dozen or so clotting factors are sequentially activated to finally convert the circulating protein fibrinogen to form the weblike latticework of fibers called fibrin. This web traps red blood cells circulating through it, locking them into a tightly packed jumble, which we call a blood clot. It's that red-purple scab that forms on a cut on your skin. This clot has the staying power needed to protect the injury for the duration of the initial repair process. Platelets and fibrinogen, the beginning and the end of the clotting cascade, have been found to be instrumental at every stage of the atherosclerotic process.

When a tiny injury occurs on the arterial wall, it attracts these platelets as well as our old nemesis, the LDL particles. Eventually, fibrinogen lays down a deposit of fibrin upon the arterial wall. If this fibrin is allowed to stay in place and is not dissolved by the fibrinolytic system, it becomes a major element of the initial injury repair process, and stimulates the accumulation of smooth muscle cells, which normally constitute the main cellular component of the injured artery in need of repair. At the same time,

LDL particles are also accumulating in the same place, creating a thickened, cholesterol-laden bulge where once there was a microscopic space or tear in the arterial wall lining.

The effects on this process of having a sedentary lifestyle are disastrous. Being sedentary not only gears the fibrinolytic system down but also increases fibrinogen levels which results in more circulating substance from which to form these troublesome blood clots, while the system for dissolving them is much less active. The fibrin that's been deposited upon the arterial walls stays there, stimulating the muscle cells beneath it to migrate upward and thicken the arterial wall from below while the LDL particles accumulate from above. As LDL particles accumulate within the wall of the artery, the muscle cells that form the inner layer of this wall continue their disorganized multiplication, further thickening the lesion. Eventually a cap formed from strands of fibrin and clotted blood grows over the cholesterol accumulation. And that is the beginning of atherosclerosis.

The cap then cracks, attracting more platelets and fibrinogen. The resulting additional fibrin clot just lies there. As the years pass, the process repeats itself. In addition to being sedentary our couch potato takes a smoking break, then the toxic smoke can cause a new fissure in the lesion; another layer of fibrin accumulates. Afterward, he drives to a fast-food restaurant and has a cheeseburger and fries. The resultant flood of lipids entering his bloodstream causes the cells of the coronary arterial wall, just having relaxed in recovery from the cigarette smoke, to stiffen up again as a result of the complex chemical interaction of the high concentration of oxidized fat suddenly interfacing with the endothelial cells. This stiffening distorts the structure of the stiff atherosclerotic lesion, and it cracks again. More fibrin is laid down; and each time another layer of fibrin forms, the blood flow channel narrows a little more. Eventually, the clot becomes so large it partially or completely blocks off blood flow. And that puts the victim in the emergency room. To dissolve the clot, the doctor administers a clot-dissolving drug or inserts a catheter.

It is essential to optimize your ability to dissolve all of those microclots forming in your arteries. This means you want to raise the levels or enhance the activity of the components of your fibrinolytic (clot-dissolving) system while minimizing the efficiency of your clotting system. Of course, there's a balance to be struck. You don't want to bleed either. This means managing the risk factors that promote clot formation while promoting the factors that stimulate clot dissolution.

Fibrinogen and Blood Clotting

Fibrinogen is the molecule that forms the actual strands of the web that traps the red blood cells and locks them into a clot. It also controls the viscosity of the blood. The more fibrinogen, the thicker blood becomes. And thicker blood flows less easily, especially through partially blocked passages.

Seven major well-designed studies have uniformly implicated high fibrinogen levels as a risk for cardiac disease. One study found the risk of high fibrinogen levels to be greater than that of high cholesterol levels. Fibrinogen is an accomplice, helping other risk factors do their damage through the clotting system. Smoking is a good example of this. Smoking injures artery walls, attracting fibrinogen to form clots at the injured places. High fibrinogen levels make the damage of smoking worse.

Pooling the data of the seven studies, the average increased risk found between those in the lowest and highest thirds of the fibrinogen level range was about 250%. Because of this compelling data the American College of Cardiology amended the quiz you filled out for yourself in chapter 5 to determine your individual risk by adding a multiplication factor for fibrinogen:

Fibrinogen Level	Risk	
	Male	*Female*
less than 235	– 20%	– 20%
235–335	average	average
greater than 335	+ 20%	+ 30%

Unlike many of the circulation's other risk factors, one does not have to have pathologically elevated levels of fibrinogen to incur a substantially increased risk from its presence—even the top third of the normal range carries increased risk.

Factors Associated with High Fibrinogen Levels

- Smoking
- African-American genetic background
- Male sex
- Advanced age
- Excess weight
- High carbohydrate diet
- Increased total cholesterol
- High triglycerides
- High LDL
- Low HDL
- Stress
- Menopause
- Oral contraceptives
- Genetics
- Diabetes
- Lack of exercise

Testing Fibrinogen Levels

Testing your fibrinogen level is easy and inexpensive—the hard part is getting a fibrinogen level that accurately represents your baseline. Concentrations of fibrinogen rise and fall rapidly in response to many stimuli. Psychological stress, an infection as mild as a cold, trauma large and small, can all cause fibrinogen levels to rise. Most confusingly, heart disease itself can cause fibrinogen levels to rise, so that having a high fibrinogen level is both a risk for and a symptom of cardiac illness.

So getting an accurate reading of your baseline fibrinogen level is not easy. The test must be done when you have no concurrent illness, however trivial, and no recent trauma, surgical or

111

accidental. And you can't get an accurate reading until at least six months after a heart attack.

For a person trying to prevent heart disease, fibrinogen is a predictive risk factor. For someone who already has heart disease, it is both a disease marker and a risk factor for aggravated illness. When people with active disease who have had actual heart attacks have been tested for fibrinogen, those with the higher levels not only had a much greater frequency of instability in their disease but also had dramatically increased incidences of repeat occlusion of their coronaries. This is a vicious circle: A person with a high level of fibrinogen has a higher risk for developing coronary artery disease. And a person with heart disease produces more fibrinogen, making the disease worse.

For a heart disease victim, a falling fibrinogen level in response to therapeutic interventions not specifically aimed at fibrinogen per se may be an indicator of a cooling off of the atherosclerotic process itself.

Lowering Fibrinogen Levels

Smoking is the number one elevator of fibrinogen levels. This is a dose dependent effect: the more you smoke, the higher your fibrinogen. The solution is clear: Stop smoking. Otherwise, some of the same general, behavioral interventions that are so useful in reducing lipid-related risk factors will also minimize fibrinogen levels: Weight loss to a body mass index (BMI) below 27 (see chapter 13) and regular exercise at a level of at least 2,000 calories per week have proven effective. By enhancing the fibrinolysis system exercise also dissolves the clot-forming fibrin strands that result from activation of fibrinogen. So exercise not only reduces the body's ability to produce fibrinogen but also helps remove its troublesome end results as well.

For women experiencing menopause, an elevated fibrinogen level may be another argument in favor of using estrogens in the postmenopausal period. Though most of the studies looking at fibrinogen as a risk marker have studied only men, studies have also confirmed its importance in women. A study in which angiograms were performed on 101 women found an over 300 percent risk for having a positive angiogram when fibrinogen levels were higher than 283. This is just about the middle value of

---

Factors That Lower Fibrinogen Levels

- Exercise
- Caucasian genetic background
- Female sex
- Regular alcohol consumption
- Postmenopausal hormone therapy
- Diet high in vegetables and fish oils

---

fibrinogen in the normal range of this factor in the general population.

Finally, fibrates, the same group of drugs used to lower triglycerides, have been shown to be effective in lowering fibrinogen levels as well.

Factors That Enhance Blood Clotting

Lipids

There is a powerful synergism between the clot system and lipid status. The rapid accumulation of large amounts of lipids on a lesion makes them swollen and more prone to severe ruptures, which then exposes large surface areas of lipids. Lipids exposed in this manner are the most intense of all stimuli to the clotting system. In addition, high levels of LDL cholesterol and triglycerides stimulate increased production of specific circulating clotting factors. This occurs with highly oxidized LDL particles most commonly found in LDL subclass B and Lp(a), especially in the presence of high LDL cholesterol levels.

Obesity

Obesity increases fibrinogen levels and lowers the activity of the fibrinolytic system. It also predisposes anyone to most of the other risk factors mentioned in this section.

113

Smoking

Smoking has one of the most comprehensive and deadly synergisms with the clotting mechanism. In fact, based on data from the Framingham Study, about *half* of the deleterious effect smoking has on the risk for heart disease is based on its ability to raise fibrinogen levels. Fibrinogen levels rise in a direct relation to the number of cigarettes smoked. Smoking also causes direct damage to the endothelial cells lining the arterial wall, which promotes new deposition of fibrin. Smoking enhances the ability of platelets to collect at the arterial wall and to stimulate the start of the clotting processes. Smoking causes rises in the adrenalinelike hormones called catecholamines, which can be directly toxic to the arterial endothelial cells and also increase the activity of platelets. All of the last four mechanisms can cause acute rupture of an established atherosclerotic plaque.

Stress

Stress causes surges of catecholamines. These can cause damage to the cells lining the artery or can precipitate rupture of an already established plaque by raising the velocity of blood flow and the blood pressure. Catecholamines also cause the arteries to constrict, narrowing what might already be a narrowed flow channel. This constriction of the blood vessels also deforms atherosclerotic plaque, causing it to crack.

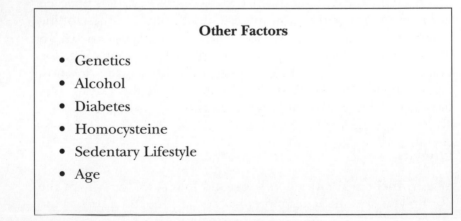

Other Factors

- Genetics
- Alcohol
- Diabetes
- Homocysteine
- Sedentary Lifestyle
- Age

Testing and Therapy of Blood-Clotting Problems

Testing your fibrinogen level is the only commonly available test that can characterize the risk your clotting system represents. Fibrinogen testing is routine and has been available for a long time. Only recently, however, has its importance with respect to heart disease been realized. In addition to this test, some people who are undergoing medical care at large medical centers can also have a few other elements of the fibrinolysis system checked by a special hematology lab. But that's about it, because testing for fibrinolytic and blood-clotting factors is otherwise difficult and imprecise.

Platelets and Aspirin

Aspirin significantly reduces the ability of platelets to stick to damaged tissue and one another, and therefore reduces their ability to form that initial plug in the clotting sequence. Aspirin prevents clumps of platelets from triggering clot formation. There's no specific test needed to see if you need aspirin.

Unless you have one of the problems mentioned, aspirin, especially in the doses required for this purpose, is an extremely safe medication. Even people with chronic stomach problems can tolerate it quite well, if they take the smallest dose in an enteric coated form; but in such cases, consult your doctor.

Who shouldn't use aspirin? Of course, anyone allergic to it cannot take it. People on anticlotting medication should not take it either. Anyone with a bleeding disorder will have to avoid it. Ulcer disease, chronic gastritis, and reflux or other inflammatory stomach problems are also contraindications. Those with poorly controlled high blood pressure or a history of brain hemorrhage or other abnormalities of cerebral circulation must also avoid it. And children should not take it either because of the danger of Reye's syndrome.

Aspirin reduces risk for a heart attack by 25 percent in people with coronary artery disease. This level of protection varies from population to population, conveying as much as a 50 percent reduction in risk in some groups. Though most of our data pertains to men, in the Nurses' Health Study of almost ninety thousand women, there was also a 25 percent reduction in heart attacks, with the benefit increasing to almost 40 percent for women over fifty.

It is very clear that aspirin reduces risk for heart attacks and is protective against second heart attacks, episodes of chest pain, and reocclusion of opened coronary arteries; in short, aspirin is a key weapon against the plaque rupture phenomenon.

Anyone with risk factors for coronary artery disease who does not have a contraindication should be on aspirin. The doses required are minute. One baby aspirin a day has been proven sufficient, and an adult 325 mg tablet is the maximum. Paradoxically, higher doses may lose the intended effect. The aspirin tablet should be coated (enteric coated aspirin), so it doesn't dissolve in the stomach and cause irritation.

12

Step Seven:
Change Your Diet Now

Everyone knows that a low-fat diet is a preventive measure against heart disease. The studies have proved it; the interpretation of the statistics is not in doubt. Yet in these same studies, anywhere from one-fifth to one-third of those tested demonstrate no benefit from a low-fat diet. Moreover, many high-risk people have cholesterol levels that don't budge regardless of how strict their diet is. The fact is that no single diet is right for everyone, so the question we have to answer is: Which diet is right for you?

Penetrating the Genome:
The Apoprotein E Gene Variants

I've saved the testing of the gene coding for the Apoprotein E for last in our discussion of blood tests for risk factors. It's not because this risk factor is any less important than the others. Quite the contrary. Unlike many of the other risk factors to which you've been introduced, the Apoprotein E gene affects everyone and is an important universal factor controlling cholesterol levels in the human population. Indeed, its variability across the spectrum of ethnic groups is one of the major reasons for different levels of susceptibility to coronary artery disease among different populations. To understand diet, you have to understand the Apoprotein E gene. Which variant of this gene you carry will suggest which diet is best for you.

Just what does this gene, or more precisely, the factor it codes for, do?

The Apoprotein E is a "pilot" protein attached to the various lipoprotein particles, including the VLDLs (very low density lipoproteins), directing them to the various stations of metabolism throughout the body's complex of metabolic highways.

How the Apoprotein E works to influence total cholesterol, LDL and HDL cholesterol, and triglycerides is extraordinarily complex and not well understood. But we do have at least part of the picture. Apoprotein E attaches to the VLDL particle that emerges from the liver. A mix of cholesterol and triglyceride molecules, this VLDL particle is transformed into the troublesome LDL and IDL particles. The Apoprotein E gene can assume three different forms numbered 2, 3, and 4. Each number designates a variant of the gene; each variant produces a slightly differently structured Apoprotein E.

Lipid particles that aren't consumed by cells or deposited in the various tissues of the body circulate back to the liver to be metabolized and either discarded or recirculated. Apoprotein E aids in this process. When the Apoprotein E gene creates the Apoprotein E variant with the number 4, or E4, it causes increased accumulation of these particles in the liver, which then stimulates a feedback mechanism that shuts down any further activity. In a sense, the E4 gene shuts down the cholesterol-absorbing properties of the liver, leaving cholesterol to accumulate in your arteries.

Worse, the E4 gene also enhances gut absorption of fat. So when an E4 person eats fat, it is absorbed quickly. The liver again gets bloated with the rush of fats into it and shuts down its ability to process the lipids, pumping more of them back into the circulation. So the E4 person's net lipid particle levels are very sensitive to fat in the diet.

Another variant of the Apoprotein E gene is numbered 2, or E2. This variant does not stimulate the liver to stop processing lipids, so the steady flow of lipid particles back into the liver never stops. The result is that they are much more efficiently cleared from the bloodstream.

The E2 person can eat a lot of fat and cholesterol, and it just gets cleared from the circulation. This increased clearance is aided by the fact that the fat in the digestive tract of an E2 is also absorbed more slowly. The E2, unlike the E4, is insensitive to changes in the amount of fat in the diet. When his diet is changed from a "normal" diet, which is 30 to 40 percent fat, to a high-carbohydrate diet that is under 30 percent fat, the E2 person will see little change in his cholesterol level, and his triglyceride levels may be significantly raised.

The E3 (the most common type) is somewhere in between the two extremes of efficiency at clearing lipids, usually dropping cholesterol levels about half as much as their E4 counterparts in response to a low-fat diet.

The effect of the low-fat diet in Apoprotein E4 and E3 people is to reduce LDL cholesterol levels by reducing the number of large LDL A particles. But they don't disappear. They become smaller, shifting the distribution of LDL particles toward the small, dense B range. This shift isn't enough to change such people from subclass A to subclass B, but for certain people, as we will see, it may have important treatment implications.

There are two genes available for every trait. This means that a person can have any one of six combinations of the Apoprotein E gene: 2/2; 3/2; 3/3; 2/4; 3/4; and 4/4.* Any combination containing 4 is associated with increased total and LDL cholesterol levels and higher Apoprotein B or LDL particle number levels. The 2/2 and 2/3 people have lower levels of these factors, with the 3/3 people falling in between. Risk parallels these lipid values: The 4/4 individual has about a 30 percent increased risk over the 3/3 person, who represents the "average" risk, and about a 60 percent increased risk versus the 3/2 and 2/2 people. The 3/4 person has an increased risk somewhere between 15 and 20 percent compared to the "average" 3/3 person.

Relative Frequencies of Apoprotein E Types in Populations

2/2	3/2	3/3	2/4	3/4	4/4
1%	10%	62%	2%	20%	5%

---

*There is little data on the Apoprotein E 4/2 person mainly because it's such a rare type. Though more common than the 2/2 type, 2/2s have a predictable response pattern because it's a "pure" type. The 4/2 person represents a hybrid of two contradictory forms of the gene. My approach with such a person therefore is similar to the 3/3 person: trial and error.

One person in four will respond very favorably to a low-fat diet, while about one in ten definitely won't and might even become worse. That leaves about 60 percent of the population with a question mark. On the basis of the Apoprotein E test we can't predict which among these Apoprotein E 3/3 people will respond favorably to a low-fat diet or how good the response will be. One can only adopt the diet and see.

The Apoprotein E2 Problem

People with the Apoprotein E2 variant get elevated triglyceride levels in response to a low-fat diet. Only 1 percent of the population has the E2/2 combination. This is fortunate because these people are in a very real sense a dormant bomb. What can ignite them? A low-fat, high-carbohydrate diet!

Normally these people are at the lowest risk for coronary artery disease on the Apoprotein E spectrum, but such a diet causes an explosion of triglycerides. This is the condition referred to in medicine as Type III hyperlipidemia, and carries an extraordinary risk, once unleashed, for coronary artery disease because of excess production of IDL particles. But unlike the rare E2/2 variant, there are many people with the E3/2 variant—I'm one of them. Since high-carbohydrate diets in these people will also cause relative elevations in triglycerides, declines in HDL, and no change in LDL, there's no benefit for them in such a diet.

Apoprotein E and HDL

This issue is much less understood, but we do know that the Apoprotein E4 is associated with demonstrably impaired reverse cholesterol transport. In the E4 person, these HDL particles seem to get "clogged up" with the cholesterol and are unable to unload it, slowing up the reverse cholesterol transport cycle.

This is the baseline condition when the Apoprotein E4 person is on a "regular" fat diet. A low-fat diet might mildly reduce HDL cholesterol and HDL2 levels unless some behavioral counterforce, like exercise, is exerted at the same time to counter this. The Apoprotein E3 and E4 people (that is, 3/3, 3/4, 4/4) follow this pattern without great differences among them. The situation with the Apoprotein E 3/2 and 2/2 people is different, however. The Apoprotein E2 variant causes not only a more severe decrease in total HDL in response to a low-fat diet but also a shift to a smaller, more ineffective HDL particle type. This is probably the result of these particles acquiring high levels of triglycerides and becoming smaller and more dense. Reverse cholesterol transport is thus impaired. So while low-fat diets may have a mildly deleterious effect on HDL levels for the E3 and E4 people, they can be disastrous for the E2.

The Importance of Determining Your Apoprotein E Type

Apoprotein E4 constitutes an independent risk factor for coronary artery disease. And you can't change your Apoprotein E status; it is in your genes.

What you can do is use it to guide you in choosing a healthful diet. With regard to LDL and HDL levels:

• The Apoprotein E 3/4 and 4/4 person on a low-fat diet will reduce LDL cholesterol twice as much as an Apoprotein E 3/3 on the same diet. The reduction of HDL levels will be mild if it occurs at all.

• The Apoprotein E 3/3 person may have a modestly beneficial response to a low-fat diet, or may have no response. HDL levels may stay the same or decline.

• The Apoprotein E 2/3 person will probably have no response to the low-fat diet and may get worse because of rising LDL levels, seriously falling HDL levels, or both.

• The Apoprotein E 2/2 person should never be placed on a low-fat diet.

Many commercial laboratories around the country are equipped to provide this test, and everyone concerned with risk for heart disease and contemplating a major change in diet should get it. It is even more important for people with a positive family history or those planning a weight reduction diet. And those with multiple risk factors for coronary artery disease or who have active disease should absolutely find out their Apoprotein E status.

LDL Subclass and Your Diet

Your LDL subclassification is much more than just a statement about the structure and activity of your LDL particles. It describes how you process the food you eat. The orientations of the metabolic pathways that process the nutrients streaming in from the digestive tract are determined by the same genes that determine LDL subclass. Their impact on how you respond to fundamental changes in your diet have been found to be even *more* powerful than the influence exerted by the Apoprotein E gene—about twice as powerful.

In addition, the effects of LDL subclass on diet response can be contrary to those of the Apoprotein E gene. In such a situation, the subclass effect will win out, but it will be blunted by the contrary stimulus. Conversely, where the two predispose to the same response, their effects will be mutually reinforcing.

Subclass A versus B

Generally, the subclass B metabolism delivers a powerful and rewarding response to a diet of less than 30 percent fat. This level of response is fairly predictable. In studies where subclass A and B men were placed on diets that were less than 30 percent fat, the subclass Bs dropped their LDL cholesterol levels by about 30 mg. In contrast, the subclass As dropped their LDL cholesterol by only 10 to 15 mg.

In response to a less than 30 percent fat diet, the subclass B person will experience a drastic drop in the largest LDL particles, the A particles and the troublesome B particles, causing a fall not just in LDL cholesterol levels but also in the number of LDL particles themselves. Thus, your Apoprotein B level, the measure of the *number* of particles, also falls. This double benefit is a major, synergistic reduction in coronary artery disease risk.

The subclass A person is different. First, only about one-third to one-half of subclass As will demonstrate a noticeable response to a low-fat diet. That response will often be a modest drop of LDL cholesterol of about 10 mg. Furthermore, the LDL particles that fall in the subclass A person are almost exclusively the big A particles.

Investigators were shocked that about 40 percent of subclass A men given a low-fat diet experienced so severe a shift in LDL particle sizes that they actually converted from subclass A to subclass B. In effect, 40 percent of the subclass A men studied actually increased their risk for heart disease as a result of the low-fat diet!

The tip-off that this was happening was that in the subclass As *who changed* to subclass Bs, triglycerides increased significantly, usually about 60 mg. This 60-mg rise in triglyceride was also seen in the subclass B people, but for unknown reasons it did not affect LDL particles in this group.

What about Women?

There are fewer studies of women that explore the issue of diet and LDL subclass interactions. This time the reason isn't neglect, however; it's just that while 35 percent of the male population are subclass Bs, only about 12 percent of premenopausal women are. There is, however, some very sobering information about women's responses to diet changes.

Most young women are LDL subclass A, but their response to a low-fat diet will be determined by genetics. Unlike men, women do not necessarily respond to diet as a subclass A. How they respond will be determined by the LDL subclass of their parents. Women with one or two subclass A parents had an average 7-mg drop in LDL cholesterol levels when their diets were changed from 35 percent to 20 percent fat. This isn't very impressive, representing a small improvement in risk. As with subclass A men, the major change was a drop in large LDL particles, with a shifting in distribution toward smaller particles. Again, as with men, a significant number of subclass A women shifted over to the B category and, therefore, didn't benefit at all from the low-fat diet.

In women whose parents were both subclass B, the response to the diet change was very much like that seen in overt subclass

B men: drastic falls in LDL cholesterol—more than five times that of the women with one or two subclass A parents, with the decrease mainly in the *small* LDL particles. These people had major improvements in risk. The reason for this is the pre-menopausal state and the hormone estrogen. It has the power to stop the subclass B genes from determining your LDL particle characteristics. However, it does *not* have the power to block the myriad other metabolic responses also associated with those genes. So women, when contemplating a low-fat diet, should look at their parents. Your response may be dictated more by *their* LDL subclass status than your own.

Combining Apoprotein E and LDL Subclass Information

You can now see how two powerful genetic factors regulate the way you metabolize fats. The effects of your Apoprotein E gene variant and your LDL subclass status can be either competitive or reinforcing on both your LDL *and* HDL levels.

LDL and HDL Response to Low-Fat Diet (<30% Fat)

Group	LDL Response	Total HDL Response	HDL Subclass Response
Subclass A	variable	reduced levels	unfavorable
Subclass B	reduced levels	reduced levels	neutral
Apo E2*	variable	reduced levels	unfavorable
Apo E3*	variable	reduced levels	neutral
Apo E4*	reduced levels	reduced levels	neutral

*Note: E2 includes only E 2/3 people. E 2/2 people should *not* be on low-fat diets. E3 includes 3/3 only. E4 includes 3/4 and 4/4 people.
If a reduction in HDL cholesterol occurs, check your HDL subclasses. Often the HDL2 is unaffected or may even rise, while the HDL3 fraction falls. It is the HDL2 that is considered the more protective.

The LDL effects depicted in the table add up. That means that if a "variable" LDL response is added to a "reduced" response, the effect will be to reduce risk modestly. If on the other hand, two "reduced" responses are combined, the subsequent reduction will be very great.

Interpreting HDL effects is much more complicated. In almost all people a low-fat, high-carbohydrate diet will cause a reduction of total HDL cholesterol levels. However, that reduced level may not adversely affect risk or detract from the benefits of the associated reduction in LDL levels. You can see this in your total cholesterol/HDL ratio. A falling ratio means more benefit is being derived from the reduction in LDL. A rising ratio might imply a problem. Another check is to see if the more protective HDL2 subclass percentage has fallen. That, too, would be an undesirable result of a diet.

Subclass Bs enjoy the benefit of a low-fat diet without some of the unfavorable side effects. Apoprotein E2 people, as well as many of the E3s, might be better off on a "normal" fat diet.

Though this table is helpful as a guide, it's just a statistical generalization, providing you with the most likely result for your situation. Not all subclass A people will have unfavorable HDL responses, and not all subclass B people will have more benign responses.

In the following table, I've listed the possible six combinations of Apoprotein E variant and LDL subclass to show what the net effect of reducing fat will probably be. This guide should be used to determine initially which diet is best for you.

Suggested Combinations of LDL Subclass and Apoprotein E

LDL Subclass	Apoprotein E	Desirable Percentage of Fat in Diet
A	E2	"normal" fat: 30–40%
A	E3	variable: start with 30%
A	E4	low fat: 25–30%
B	E2	low fat or variable: start with 30%
B	E3	low fat: 25–30% (may need "normal" fat)
B	E4	low fat: 25–30%

Tracking Diet Response in Subclass A

Don't expect overnight changes. It takes at least six weeks to two months of honestly following your new diet to begin to see results. The right person on the right diet can enjoy 30- to 40-mg reductions of LDL levels. It's been shown that in populations where LDL cholesterol levels represent the predominant risk factor, a 1 percent reduction of LDL cholesterol levels yields an impressive 2 percent reduction in risk for coronary artery disease. But of course different combinations of subclass and Apoprotein E status will have different results.

Only subclass As who have an Apoprotein E2 gene in their profile should presume they will get no benefit from the low-fat diet. On the other side of the spectrum, big benefits can almost be guaranteed for the subclass A people who have an Apoprotein E4 gene. For those in between—most subclass A people—the low-fat diet is definitely worth trying, but close monitoring is absolutely crucial. There is a tradeoff: You could end up reducing large A particles without reducing total LDL. This means an increase in more malignant smaller-size LDL particles. So you wind up lowering your risk with your LDL cholesterol level, but raising it with your particle distribution.

There are a number of warning signs that this may be happening. After six to eight weeks on a new diet, let's assume your LDL cholesterol level has fallen somewhat. The Apoprotein B test can detect if that fall indicates a reduction in particle number or just a shift in particle type. Any large positive shifts in the Apoprotein B/LDL cholesterol ratio should be a warning sign, and a shift to a ratio of 1.1 or greater is a reason to recheck your LDL subclass status. If the ratio of Apoprotein B to LDL cholesterol has risen above 1.1, there is even a good chance you've shifted into the subclass B state, worsening your situation. This is an indication to get off that diet and go to a diet more in the range of 30 to 40 percent fat. Some people may see declines in both LDL cholesterol and Apo B levels. That's the most desirable situation but also unfortunately the most uncommon. But if this happens, you're on the right diet.

Triglycerides and Subclass A

Low-fat, high-carbohydrate diets can increase triglyceride levels. As far as we know, triglycerides themselves are not a risk factor promoting plaque formation, so this in itself may not be a problem. The problem is that triglycerides alter the structure and activity of the other lipid particles, and lipid particles do promote plaque formation.

In the studies where subclass As got in trouble with the low-fat diet, the triglycerides rose by variable amounts. While as a whole, the population of A and B subjects demonstrated about a 40-mg rise in triglycerides, the subclass As who remained subclass As increased their triglycerides by about 20 mgs, whereas those subclass As who converted to Bs boosted their triglycerides by about 45.

A rise in triglycerides on a high-carbohydrate, low-fat diet is to be expected. It's when these rises are substantial, about 40 or more, that LDL subclass status should be checked.

HDL and Subclass A

Low-fat diets almost uniformly cause HDL levels to fall, especially in the subclass A person, an average of about 18 percent. Even worse, there can be a decrease in the percentage of the protective HDL2 subfraction, thus further intensifying the adverse effects of the diet.

So are you better off or worse off on a low-fat diet? If the fall in your LDL and HDL cholesterol levels results in a higher total cholesterol/HDL cholesterol ratio, you haven't done yourself any good. If the ratio remains unchanged, you should check your HDL subclass test.

The following table summarizes current information about what happens when you're on a low-fat diet, and what you should do about it.

Falling Apoprotein B/LDL cholesterol ratio	Desirable
Rising Apoprotein B/LDL cholesterol ratio	Caution
Apoprotein B/LDL cholesterol ratio greater than 1.1	Check LDL subclass
Rise in triglyceride levels of about 50	Check LDL subclass
LDL subclass A changes to B	Go back to "normal" fat diet
Falling total cholesterol/HDL ratio	Desirable
Stable total cholesterol/HDL ratio (when HDL cholesterol is in "average" range)	Check HDL2 percentage (should not fall)

Tracking Diet Response in Subclass B

Generally, it's the subclass B person who will respond best to the low-fat diet. This is true across the spectrum of Apoprotein E gene types (exception: Apoprotein E2/2s have no LDL subclass and should avoid such diets). If one is an Apoprotein E3/2, it is worth trying a low-fat diet, but your level of monitoring should be the same as if you were a subclass A: you need to check your HDLs, triglycerides, and total cholesterol/HDL ratio after six to eight weeks on the diet.

With the above exception, subclass B people on a low-fat diet will have substantial decreases in LDL cholesterol levels, and many of the specific particles disappearing will be just the ones you want to get rid of—the small dense troublemakers.

HDL and Subclass B

HDLs fall on the low-fat diet, but the total cholesterol/HDL ratio improves, thanks to a much greater drop in LDL levels. Moreover, the HDL particles that vanish are mostly the less important HDL3 particles, and the number of more protective HDL2 particles is preserved.

Triglycerides and Subclass B

The major factor the subclass B person on a low-fat diet needs to watch is triglyceride level. Invariably, it rises, and the rises can be substantial, typically around 60 mgs or so. This usually doesn't cause a problem. For some reason, when the subclass B person responds to a low-fat diet, the rise in triglycerides does not affect the fall in small dense LDL particles and Apoprotein B levels.

However, very high increases in triglyceride levels can cause problems for some subclass B people. Their HDL cholesterol levels may fall too much and/or the HDL particle profile may change and shift to smaller dense HDL particles in the HDL3 range.

Low HDL levels, rising total cholesterol/HDL ratios, or average HDL levels with falling HDL2 percentages are all indications that although you've had a great response in reducing the amount of LDL cholesterol and number of LDL particles, triglycerides have become too high and are causing problems. This is when the high-carbohydrate, low-fat diet may need to be more carefully scrutinized and modified by either changing the nature of the carbohydrates being eaten, or eating more of specific kinds of fats.

With these considerations in mind, let's now turn to what exactly a low-fat, high-carbohydrate diet should look like.

Proper Diet Composition and the Problem of the Low-Fat Diet

Not all low-fat diets are alike. And the improper construction of the "heart-healthy" diet is as often the reason for poor metabolic responses as is any inherent intolerance on the part of a particular individual.

One of the problems associated with low-fat diets is their effects on HDL and LDL particles. Lack of fat and the overabundance of carbohydrates are both independent and synergistic factors. On average, HDL levels drop 10 percent for every 10 percent rise in the amount of energy provided by carbohydrate rather than fat.

The almost universally accepted dietary guidelines that advise lowering fat to anywhere between 30 and 10 percent of total calories can be very counterproductive if they don't result in substantial reductions in LDL levels. So the problem is to design a low-fat diet that reduces LDLs while preserving HDLs.

First, let's look at increased carbohydrates. When researchers examine exactly what people eat on a low-fat diet, they find that 20 percent or so of the added carbohydrates provided to replace the fat calories were *sugar*. For many of us, this is not helpful. When you eat an inappropriately high sugar load, this large delivery of sugar gets dumped into your bloodstream, sending insulin levels surging. But if the sugar load is just too great for that corresponding surge to handle or the cells just don't want it, the extra sugar gets returned to the liver, which converts it to triglycerides. Now you have a spillage of triglycerides into the bloodstream. The increased triglyceride concentration and surges of insulin adversely affect lipid particles.

129

But if you substitute big, long-chained, difficult-to-digest car-bohydrates like the starches found in whole grains and unprocessed rice, this dumping phenomenon doesn't occur, and the triglyceride levels don't shoot up. In most cases, they will rise somewhat, but not as they would with sugar.

The American version of the high-carbohydrate, low-fat diet is not the rice and beans, potatoes and barley diets of other coun-tries. Instead, we replace our fats with sweetened yogurt, baked goods made of highly refined flour, sugar-coated breakfast cere-als, low-fat cookies, and no-fat cakes. And even the more thought-ful among us who smugly shun such foods as we're eating a what-could-be-healthier bowl of fruit are falling into the trap: eating more simple sugar.

This brings us to an unexpected solution: fat. Believe it or not, the solution lies in carefully and methodically substituting at least some of those carbohydrates with fat. But not just any fat.

Fats

When you think of fat, you're really thinking of triglycerides, triplets of fatty acids connected to a glycerol molecule. This is the fat we're talking about when we talk about fat as an energy source. Based on their molecular structure, these fats can be divided into saturated and unsaturated types.

Monounsaturated Fats

Researchers studying heart attack risk in Europe noticed some-thing very odd about the geographical distribution of risk. For some reason, the E4 variant of the Apoprotein E gene, which in most parts of Europe means an increased risk for heart disease, seems to lose its power in populations that inhabit the Mediterranean basin. The gene is still there, but it doesn't seem to assert itself. We now believe that one of the reasons for this powerful resistance to atherosclerosis is something people in the Mediterranean have in their diet in abundance: olive oil. Where more olive oil is consumed, the risk for heart disease declines. Calorie for calorie, olive oil is the most concentrated source of monounsaturated fat in nature and the most efficient delivery system for it:

Sources of Monounsaturated Fats
(1 tbsp = 120 calories/14 grams of fat)

Oil	Percentage of Mono	1 tbsp Mono Grams	1 tbsp Mono Calories	1 tbsp Total Calories
olive	77%	11	96	120
canola	58%	8	73	120
peanut*	48%	7	60	120
fish oil	30%	4	38	120
nut oils	variable 12–30%	—	—	120
avocado puree (or oil)	65%	12	108	185
½ cup (18 g fat)	(of fats)	(½ cup)	(½ cup)	(½ cup)

*Also has high saturated fat.

Monounsaturated fats, when substituted for saturated fats, may allow one's HDL levels, which may have been depressed by a high-carbohydrate diet, to recover by 50 to as much as 100 percent *without* a corresponding rise in LDL cholesterol levels.

In addition, monounsaturated fats don't make triglycerides rise. They hit the problem of the adverse effects of too much sugar both ways. First, they provide fat for regeneration of HDL levels without providing fuel for production of more LDL particles. And as an added bonus, they help stabilize the LDL particle against becoming oxidized, which is so important in preventing the atherosclerotic process from progressing.

Monounsaturated fats, like complex carbohydrates, are not a panacea. They are, after all, fat, and fat means they pack 9 calories per gram versus 4 calories per gram of carbohydrate or protein. Furthermore, that calorie-dense effect is amplified by about another 25 percent because it takes very little energy to metabolize a calorie of fat compared to carbohydrates. In effect then, any fat, including mono and the omega-3s (discussed later) effectively delivers about *11* calories per gram when compared to the four calories per gram of carbohydrates. There's no advantage in substituting monos for carbohydrates if it's going to result in a weight gain.

**Those Who Benefit Most
from High Monounsaturated Diets**

subclass B

high Lp(a)

smokers

low HDL

triglycerides > 200

subclass A with coronary artery disease

diabetics

So how do you safely convert carbohydrate calories in your diet to monos? For every gram of carbohydrate, or every 4 calories of carbohydrate in your diet that you wish to substitute with monounsaturated fat, the energy equivalent to your body is one-third of a gram of fat, or 3 calories.

One tablespoon of olive oil is the energy equivalent of 38 grams of carbohydrate. In the chart below, you can see what this translates into in terms of real foods.

Exchange Choices
Serving Sizes of High-Carbohydrate Food Sources
Approximately Equivalent to 1 Tablespoon Olive Oil

	Serving Size
Bagel	
cinnamon raisin	¾ bagel
plain	¾ bagel
Barley Flakes, pearled, dry measure	1½ oz
Barley, cooked	¾ cup
Biscuit, Healthy Valley Buttermilk	¾ biscuit
Bread	
fresh baked, white	2 slices
fresh baked, white, low calorie	2½ slices
Arnold, wheat	2 slices
Arnold, Italian light	3 slices
Arnold, brick oven white	2½ slices

	Serving Size
Oatmeal Goodness	2 slices
Pepperidge Farm, hearty country white	1½ slices
Sahara, pita	1 pita
Wonder, rye	2 slices
Wonder, whole wheat	2 slices

Buckwheat

dry measure	¼ cup
groats, cooked	1 cup

Bulgur, cooked   1 cup

Cereals, Hot

Arrowhead Mills, oat bran	1⅓ oz
Arrowhead Mills, wheat	1½ oz
Cream of Wheat, instant wheat	1½ oz
H-O, instant oatmeal and oats	1 packet
H-O, instant wheat	1 packet
Quaker Oats, instant oatmeal	1 oz
Health Valley, natural oat bran	1½ oz

Cereals, Read to Eat

Arrowhead Mills, bran flakes	1½ cup
Arrowhead Mills, corn flakes	1 cup
Arrowhead Mills, puffed rice	1⅔ cup
Arrowhead Mills, puffed wheat	1⅔ cup
General Mills, Cheerios	1⅔ cup
General Mills, Count Chocula	1⅓ cup
General Mills, Fiber One	1¼ cup
General Mills, Golden Grahams	1 cup
General Mills, Honey Nut Cheerios	1 cup
General Mills, Kix	2 cups
General Mills, raisin oat bran	1 cup
General Mills, Total	1½ cup
General Mills, Wheaties	1½ cup
Kellogg's Corn Flakes	1⅓ cup
Kellogg's Frosted Flakes	1 cup
Kellogg's, Just Right	1 cup
Kellogg's, low fat granola without raisins	⅓ cup
Kellogg's, Product 19	1⅓ cup
Kellogg's, raisin bran	1 cup
Kellogg's Rice Krispies	1 cup
Nabisco, shredded wheat	1 cup
Post, Alpha-Bits	1 cup
Post, Fruit & Fibre	¾ cup
Post, Grape-Nuts	1½ cup
Quaker, Cap'n Crunch	1 cup
Quaker, Life	1 cup
Quaker, Oat'Mmms	1⅓ cup

continues

Exchange Choices *Continued*

	Serving Size
Cereals, Ready to Eat *Continued*	
Quaker, puffed rice	3 cups
Ralston, muesli	½ cup
Wheat Chex	1 cup
Corn Grits	¼ cup
Cornmeal	
degermed	¼ cup
whole grain	¼ cup
Cornstarch	¼ cup
Couscous	¾ cup
Farina, whole grain	1⅓ cup
Flour	
buckwheat	1⅓ cup
carob	⅓ cup
corn	⅓ cup
rye, dark	⅓ cup
rye, light	⅓ cup
triticale	⅓ cup
Arrowhead Mills, millet	½ cup
rice	¼ cup
Arrowhead Mills, oat	1½ oz
whole wheat	⅓ cup
Noodles	
Plain	1⅓ oz
Spinach	1⅓ oz
Oat, whole grain	½ cup
Oat Flakes	⅓ cup
Oat Groats	1⅓ oz
Pancake	
Aunt Jemima, low fat	3½ cakes
Pillsbury, Hungry Jack, original	2 cakes
Pancakes and Waffle	
Aunt Jemima, buttermilk	3⅔, 4″ cakes
Aunt Jemima, whole wheat	2¾, 4″ cakes
Pasta	
corn	1½ oz
durum Wheat	1½ oz
protein fortified	1½ oz
spinach	1½ oz
whole wheat	1½ oz
Potato Starch	¼ cup

	Serving Size
Rice Cake, plain	3¾ cake
Rice	
brown	¾ cup
basmati	1 cup
white	½ cup
Rye Cakes, Quaker, grain cakes	4¼ cakes
Rye Halves, Arrowhead Mills	1½ oz
Rye, Whole Grain	¼ cup
Semolina, Whole Grain	¼ cup
Wheat Cake, Quaker Grain Cakes	4½ cakes
Wheat Flakes, Arrowhead Mills	⅓ cup
Wheat Pilaf	¾ cup
Wheat, whole grain	¼ cup

The following two charts are valuable in helping control the amount of sugar in your diet. Listed are many of the most common foods people turn to when adopting "low-fat" diets. Many of these foods have too much sugar. Pick the foods with less than 25 percent of calories from sugar.

Sugar Content of Common "Low-Fat" Carbohydrate Sources

Item	Calories per Serving	% Total Calories as Sugar	% Total Carbohydrates as Sugar
Baked Beans			
B & M	170	19	26
Bush's Best	150	13	17
Grandma Brown's	160	7.5	11
Canned Foods			
Libby's			
lite sliced peaches	60	80	92
chunky mixed fruit	60	80	86
fruit cocktail	60	80	73
Cereal Bars			
Betty Crocker Sweet Rewards			
double fudge brownie	100	60	60
fruit variety	120	60	62
chocolate chip	110	58	70

continues

Sugar Content of Common "Low-Fat" Carbohydrate Sources *Continued*

Item	Calories per Serving	% Total Calories as Sugar	% Total Carbohydrates as Sugar
Nature's Choice			
strawberry	110	47	48
raspberry	110	47	48
blueberry	110	51	52
apple	110	51	52
SnackWell's			
apple cinnamon	120	53	55
mixed berry	130	40	50
strawberry	120	57	59
blueberry	120	50	52
raspberry	120	54	55
strawberry/banana	120	57	59
Sunbelt			
strawberry	130	55	64
blueberry	130	52	61
raspberry	130	55	64
Granola Bars			
Nature Valley			
apple brown sugar	110	25	32
honey nut	110	25	32
oatmeal	110	29	36
raisin	110	29	36
Quaker			
s'mores	110	36	45
chocolate chunk	110	36	45
chocolate chip	120	30	43
cookies n'cream	110	33	41
strawberry blast	110	40	48
SnackWell's			
fudge dipped	120	43	59
oatmeal raisin	110	50	63
caramel	120	43	59
Cakes			
Freihofer's			
banana loaf	140	57	61
chocolate loaf	120	60	62
golden loaf	130	52	61
lemon twist	130	46	52
raspberry twist	140	54	59

Item	Calories per Serving	% Total Calories as Sugar	% Total Carbohydrates as Sugar
Cookies			
Archway			
oatmeal raspberry	100	52	57
oatmeal raisin	100	56	58
cinnamon honey gems	100	52	57
devil food chocolate drop	60	60	60
molasses	90	49	58
fruit bar	90	49	52
Nabisco			
peach apricot cobblers	70	57	59
apple cinnamon cobblers	70	57	59
Fig newtons	100	56	64
Apple Newtons	100	60	65
Strawberry Newtons	100	60	65
Cranberry Newtons	100	56	63
Raspberry Newtons	100	52	57
Nilla wafers	120	40	50
SnackWell's			
creme sandwich	110	36	48
chocolate sandwich	110	40	55
double chocolate chip	130	31	48
chocolate chip	130	31	45
peanut butter chip	120	30	45
fudge brownie bar	130	52	65
chocolate cherry brownie	130	46	56
banana snack bar	130	49	59
devil food cookies cakes	50	72	75
golden devil food cake	50	64	67
Crackers			
Keebler			
graham crackers—cinnamon	110	33	38
graham crackers—honey	120	30	36
Nabisco			
cinnamon grahams	110	36	42
honey grahams	110	29	35
SnackWell's			
french onion	120	7	8
zesty cheese	120	7	9
wheat	60	13	17
classic golden	60	13	18
cracked pepper	60	7	8
Italian ranch	120	7	9
salsa cheddar	120	7	9

continues

Sugar Content of Common "Low-Fat" Carbohydrate Sources *Continued*

Item	Calories per Serving	% Total Calories as Sugar	% Total Carbohydrates as Sugar
Yogurt			
Breyers light			
cherry chocolate	130	58	83
black cherry jubilee	240	68	87
cherry vanilla cream	130	55	82
raspberry n' cream	130	55	82
blueberries n' cream	130	58	83
key lime pie	130	52	77
berry banana split	130	55	82
lemon chiffon	130	55	82
peaches n' cream	130	58	83
Breyers, 99% fat free			
black cherry parfait	240	68	87
classic strawberry	230	68	87
raspberries n' cream	230	70	87
blueberries n' cream	240	67	85
peaches n' cream	240	67	87
Columbo, light			
strawberry/banana	100	40	63
white chocolate raspberry	100	40	63
creamy vanilla	100	40	63
key lime pie	100	40	63
strawberry	100	40	63
raspberry	100	40	63
Columbo, classic			
black cherry parfait	200	72	84
cherry	200	72	84
raspberry	200	72	84
peach	200	72	84
raspberry peach melba	200	72	84
lemon	170	68	85
white chocolate raspberry	200	72	84
vanilla caramel sundae	200	82	87
Crowley, nonfat			
peach	100	40	59
banana cream	100	40	59
cappuccino	100	40	59
strawberry	100	40	59
lemon	100	40	59
raspberry	100	40	59

Item	Calories per Serving	% Total Calories as Sugar	% Total Carbohydrates as Sugar
Dannon, lite			
blueberry	100	40	59
banana cream	100	36	56
strawberry banana	100	40	63
coconut cream pie	100	36	60
mint chocolate cream pie	100	36	60
vanilla	100	36	60
cappuccino	100	36	56
raspberry	100	40	63
cherry vanilla	100	48	67
Dannon, low fat			
cherry	240	73	98
orange	240	73	98
raspberry	240	72	96
strawberry banana	240	72	96
blueberry	240	73	96
peach	240	73	98
mixed berries	240	72	96
lemon	240	58	97
plain	110	58	100
SnackWell's			
mint chocolate cheesecake	170	68	76
double chocolate	190	63	73
chocolate cherry	190	63	73
mint chocolate caramel nut	170	68	76
milk chocolate peanut butter	180	58	72
milk chocolate almond	170	68	76

Breakfast Cereals as a Carbohydrate Source
How They Compare in Sugar Content

Brand	Product Name
Cereals Less Than 15% Fat, 25% Sugar	
Arrowhead Mills	amaranth flakes
Arrowhead Mills	apple corns
Arrowhead Mills	bran flakes
Arrowhead Mills	corn flakes
Arrowhead Mills	Crispy Puffs
Arrowhead Mills	kamut flakes

continues

Breakfast Cereals as a Carbohydrate Source
Continued

Brand	Product Name
Cereals Less Than 15% Fat, 25% Sugar Continued	
Arrowhead Mills	Maple Corns
Arrowhead Mills	multigrain flakes
Arrowhead Mills	Nature O's
Arrowhead Mills	puffed corn
Arrowhead Mills	puffed kamut
Arrowhead Mills	puffed millet
Arrowhead Mills	puffed rice
Arrowhead Mills	puffed wheat
Arrowhead Mills	spelt flakes
Arrowhead Mills	wheat bran
Arrowhead Mills	wheat germ
Familia	muesli
Featherweight	corn flakes
Featherweight	crisp rice
General Mills	Basic 4
General Mills	Country Corn Flakes
General Mills	Crispy Wheats'n Raisins
General Mills	Fiber One
General Mills	Golden Grahams
General Mills	Kaboom
General Mills	Kix
General Mills	Lucky Charms
General Mills	raisin oat bran
General Mills	S'mores Grahams
General Mills	Total, mixed grain
General Mills	Total, raisin bran
General Mills	Triples, mixed grain
General Mills	Wheaties
Health Valley	10 bran O's with almonds
Health Valley	10 bran O's with apple and cinnamon
Health Valley	10 bran O's with high fiber
Health Valley	fat free granola with dates and almonds
Health Valley	fat free granola with raisins and cinnamon
Health Valley	fat free granola with sprouts and raisins
Health Valley	fat free granola with tropical fruit
Health Valley	rice bran O's
Health Valley	100% natural bran with apples and cinnamon
Health Valley	100% natural bran with raisins
Health Valley	fiber 7 flakes, mixed grain
Health Valley	flakes, bran and raisins
Health Valley	flakes, oat bran
Health Valley	flakes, oat bran with almond and dates

Brand	Product Name
Health Valley	flakes, oat bran with raisins
Health Valley	fruit & fitness, mixed grain, fruit
Health Valley	fruit lites, corn and fruit
Health Valley	fruit lites, wheat and fruit
Health Valley	health O's, mixed grain
Health Valley	lites, puffed corn
Health Valley	lites, puffed rice
Health Valley	lites, puffed wheat
Health Valley	lites, rice
Health Valley	organic bran, apple and cinnamon
Health Valley	organic bran, raisins
Kashi	Medley, mixed grain
Kashi	puffed, mixed grain
Kellogg's	40% bran flakes
Kellogg's	All-Bran, original
Kellogg's	Apple Cinnamon Squares
Kellogg's	blueberry squares
Kellogg's	Common Sense, oat bran
Kellogg's	Common Sense, oat bran and raisins
Kellogg's	Complete, bran, wheat
Kellogg's	Corn Flakes
Kellogg's	Crispix
Kellogg's	Fruitful Bran
Kellogg's	Heartwise
Kellogg's	Just Right, fiber nuggets
Kellogg's	Just Right, fruit and nuts
Kellogg's	Product 19
Kellogg's	Rice Krispies
Kellogg's	shredded wheat
Kellogg's	Special K
Kellogg's	Healthy Choice, mixed grain and brown sugar
Kellogg's	Healthy Choice, multigrain squares and honey
Kellogg's	Nutri-grain, mixed grain, almond and raisins
Kellogg's	Nutri-grain, mixed grain, golden wheat
Kellogg's	Nutri-grain, wheat, raisins
Nabisco	shredded wheat
Nabisco	shredded wheat n bran
Nabisco	Spoon Size, mini wheat
Nature Valley	toasted oat
Post	Blueberry Morning
Post	Fruit & Fibre, peaches, raisins, and almonds
Post	fruity pebbles, rice
Post	Grape-Nuts, flakes
Post	Grape-Nuts, raisins
Post	Grape-Nuts, wheat and barley

continues

Breakfast Cereals as a Carbohydrate Source
Continued

Brand	Product Name

Cereals Less Than 15% Fat, 25% Sugar Continued

Brand	Product Name
Post	Honey Bunches of Oats, honey roasted
Post	oat flakes
Post	Toasties
Post	Toasties, corn flakes
Post	natural bran flakes, bran
Post	natural bran flakes, wheat
Quaker	cinnamon oat squares
Quaker	crunchy bran
Quaker	honey graham chex
Quaker	King Vitamin
Quaker	Life
Quaker	Oat Bran
Quaker	Oat'Mmms, toasted
Quaker	Oat Squares
Quaker	Oat'Mmms, Popeye
Quaker	puffed rice
Quaker	puffed wheat
Quaker	shredded wheat, original size
Quaker	Toasted Oatmeal
Quaker	unprocessed bran
Ralston	bran news, apple, spice or cinnamon
Ralston	corn chex
Ralston	dinersaurs
Ralston	muesli, raisins, dates, and almonds
Ralston	mueslix, dates and almonds
Ralston	multibran chex, raspberries and almonds
Ralston	rice and chex
Ralston	Sun Flakes
Ralston	wheat chex, whole grain
Sunflakes	multigrain
Sunshine	wheat, shredded
Sunshine	wheat, shredded, bite size

Cereals with less than 15% fat but 25 to 40% sugar.

Brand	Product Name
Familia	muesli, original
General Mills	Berry Berry Kix
General Mills	Honey Nut Cheerios
General Mills	Oatmeal Crisp
General Mills	Wheaties, honey gold
Kellogg's	Frosted Mini-Wheats, shredded

Brand	Product Name
Kellogg's	low fat granola, without raisins
Kellogg's	low fat granola, with raisins
Kellogg's	Mueslix, crispy blend
Kellogg's	Raisin Squares, raisin filled
Post	brannola, wheat with raisins
Post	Fruit & Fibre, dates, raisins, and walnuts
Quaker	Cap'n Crunch, deep sea
Quaker	kids favorites, frosted flakes
Quaker	low fat 100% natural, whole grain with raisins
Quaker	Oat Life, Cinnamon
Ralston	crispy mini grahams
Ralston	double chex
Ralston	frosted chex jr.
Ralston	graham chex

Cereals with less than 15% fat but more than 40% sugar.

Brand	Product Name
General Mills	Body Buddies, mixed grain
General Mills	Boo Berry, mixed grain
General Mills	Cocoa Puffs, corn
General Mills	Count Chocula, corn
General Mills	Franken Berry, mixed grain
General Mills	Hidden Treasures, corn
General Mills	Trix, mixed grain
Kellogg's	Apple Jacks
Kellogg's	Cocoa Krispies
Kellogg's	Corn Pops
Kellogg's	Frosted Flakes, Corn
Kellogg's	Frosted Krispies, rice
Kellogg's	Froot Loops
Kellogg's	honey smacks
Kellogg's	raisin bran
Kellogg's	Rice Krispies, apples and cinnamon
Post	Alpha-Bits
Post	cocoa pebbles, rice
Post	Honeycomb, corn
Post	Honeycomb, mixed grain
Post	natural, raisin bran
Quaker	Cap'n Crunch
Quaker	Cap'n Crunch, Crunch Berries
Quaker	Christmas Crunch
Quaker	kids favorites, marshmallow
Quaker	Popeye, Sweet Crunch
Quaker	Popeye, Cocoa Blasts
Quaker	Popeye, fruit curls

continues

143

Breakfast Cereals as a Carbohydrate Source
Continued

Brand	Product Name

Cereals with less than 15% fat but more than 40% sugar.

Brand	Product Name
Quaker	Popeye jeepers, crispy corn puff
Quaker	Popeye jeepers, oat
Quaker	sweet puffs
Ralston	cookie crisp, chocolate chip
Ralston	cookie crisp, vanilla wafer
Ralston	TMN turtles

Cereals with 16 to 30% fat and less than 25% sugar.

Brand	Product Name
3 Minute Brand	oatmeal and oats, raisins
3 Minute Brand	oatmeal and oats, raisins and oat bran
3 Minute Brand	quick oatmeal and oats, oat bran
3 Minute Brand	regular, oat bran
Arrowhead Mills	instant, oatmeal and oats
Arrowhead Mills	instant, oatmeal and oats, apples, dates and almonds
Arrowhead Mills	instant oatmeal and oats, cinnamon, raisins and almonds
H-O Brand	gourmet, oatmeal and oats
H-O Brand	instant, oatmeal and oats
H-O Brand	instant, oatmeal and oats, fiber
H-O Brand	super bran
Mother's	instant oat bran
Mother's	instant oatmeal
Quaker	instant oat bran
Quaker	extra oatmeal and oats
Quaker	instant oatmeal and oats
Quaker	instant oatmeal and oats, dates and walnuts
Quaker	instant oatmeal and oats, peaches and cream
Quaker	old-fashioned oats
Quaker	quick oats
Quaker	quick/old-fashioned oatmeal and oats
Quaker	Mother's oat bran
Roman Meal	multigrain, apples and cinnamon
Roman Meal	premium, oatmeal and oats, wheat, dates, and raisins
Total	instant oatmeal and oats
Total	quick
Wholesome N Hearty	oat bran

Brand	Product Name
Wholesome N Hearty	Instant oat bran, honey
Alpen	mixed grain, low fat
Alpen	mixed grain, original
Arrowhead Mills	mixed grain
Arrowhead Mills	oat bran flakes
Breadshop's	granola, blueberries and cream
Breadshop's	granola, raspberries and cream
Breadshop's	granola, strawberries and cream
Familia	champion
Familia	crunchy
Familia	mixed grain
General Mills	Cheerios, oat
General Mills	Clusters, wheat
General Mills	Oatmeal Crisp
General Mills	raisin nut bran, raisins and nuts
Health Valley	amaranth, bananas
Health Valley	amaranth, flakes
Health Valley	corn flakes, corn
Health Valley	oat bran O's
Health Valley	oat bran O's, fruit and nuts
Health Valley	rice bran with almonds
Health Valley	oat bran, almond crunch
Health Valley	oat bran, fruit Hawaiian
Health Valley	oat bran, raisins and nuts
Heartland	mixed grain, natural
Heartland	mixed grain, raisins
Kellogg's	All-Bran, extra fiber
Nabisco	100% bran
Nature Valley	100% natural, cinnamon and raisins
Post	Banana Nut Crunch
Post	Great Grains, crunch pecans
Post	Great Grains, raisin, dates, and pecans
Post	Honey Bunches of Oats, almonds
Quaker	honey graham ohs
Quaker	Kretschmer, wheat
Quaker	Kretschmer, wheat honey
Quaker	Kretschmer, wheat toasted
Quaker	Toasted Oatmeal, honey and nut
Ralston	fruit muesli, raisins, walnuts, and cranberries
Ralston	muesli, raisins, peaches, pecans
Ralston	muesli, bananas and walnuts
Ralston	muesli, cranberries and walnuts

continues

Breakfast Cereals as a Carbohydrate Source
Continued

Brand	Product Name

Cereals with 16 to 30% fat and less than 25% sugar. Continued

Ralston	muesli, peaches and pecans
Sun Country	granola, mixed grain, almonds

Cereals with 16 to 30% fat and 25 to 40% sugar.

General Mills	Cinnamon Toast Crunch, mixed grain
Quaker	Cap'n Crunch, peanut butter
Ralston	honey almond delight
Sun Country	granola, mixed grain, raisins and dates

Cereals with 16 to 30% fat and more than 40% sugar.

Quaker	Ohs, Honey Graham

Cereals with 30 to 40% fat.

Roman Meal	premium, oatmeal and oats, wheat, honey, coconut
Arrowhead Mills	mixed grain, granola, maple nut
Breadshop's	granola, oat bran
Erehorn	granola, oat, dates and nuts
Erehorn	granola, oat, maple
Erehorn	granola, oat, spiced apple
Erehorn	granola, oat, sunflower crunch
General Mills	toasted oat, oat
Heartland	mixed grain, coconut
Kellogg's	Cracklin' Oat Bran
Nature Valley	100% natural, mixed grain
Nature Valley	fruit and nut, oat
Post	hearty granola
Quaker	100% natural, mixed grain
Quaker	100% natural, mixed grain, apples and cinnamon
Quaker	100% natural, mixed grain, raisins and dates
Quaker	100% natural, oat, honey
Quaker	100% natural, oat, honey and raisins
Sun Country	mixed grain, granola with raisins
Sun Country	100% natural, mixed grain, granola with almonds
Sun Country	100% natural, mixed grain, granola with raisins & dates
Sunbelt	mixed grain, granola, fruit and nuts

1 Tablespoon of Olive Oil Equivalents for Selected Fruit
(150 Calories of Carbohydrate or Carbohydrate and Protein)

5 oz. fruit juice
½ large apple (4-inch diameter)
5 oz. applesauce (unsweetened)
½ large banana
⅔ cup cherries
19 dates
9 figs
31 grapes
⅔ of 5-inch-diameter melon
3-inch-diameter orange
⅘ cup orange slices
1⅓ , 3-inch diameter peaches
⅘ cup peach slices

When to Convert Carbohydrates to Monounsaturated Fats

Triglyceride levels become a problem when they double their baseline or exceed 200, and especially if they begin to approach the 500 range. This is an indication that LDL subclass, HDL cholesterol, and even the HDL subclasses should be rechecked because they might be changing in the wrong direction. But before undergoing the inconvenience and expense of retesting, reevaluate your low, less-than-30-percent-fat diet; is it really optimal? Are simple carbohydrates limited to less than 10 percent of the diet?

Review the Sugar Content tables beginning on page 135. Are you regularly eating or drinking the foods on that list? Also, how much fruit and fruit juice are you taking in? Unfortunately, raw fruit, though usually beneficial, can present a sugar-loading problem, especially if you're also eating plenty of sugar-laden "low-fat" snacks. But don't drop the fruit. Instead, get rid of the manufactured foods. Then if there's still a problem, eliminate fruit juices; they are after all just sugar with the flavor of the original fruit and some of the vitamins. Finally, if the problem remains, limit fruit to 10 percent of calories.

If you've gone through this checklist and still seem to have a markedly elevated triglyceride problem, check to see if any of the following has occurred:

- LDL subclass A conversion to subclass B
- Rising total cholesterol/HDL ratio
- HDL cholesterol falling below 40 for men or 50 for women
- HDL2 below 23 percent for men, 27 percent for women

Yet another very important factor to consider is that you may have hidden diabetes. This should be evaluated. If none of these are a problem, then neither are the elevated triglycerides. You're doing all right.

In a typical low-fat diet where 30 percent of calories are derived from fat, half of these calories should be from monounsaturated fats—15 percent of the diet. In the situation we're describing, you should substitute with monounsaturated fats another 10 percent of total calories previously derived from carbohydrates. In addition, you should decrease your percentage of saturated and polyunsaturated fats to minimal amounts, replacing them with monos. The best way to do this is with a calorie-for-calorie substitution with olive oil. The table of olive oil equivalents on page 147 can help you do that.

Less than 6 percent of total calories should be from saturated fats, and less than 10 percent should be from polyunsaturated fats. The rest should be monos.

One of the great conveniences of monounsaturated fats not shared by any of the other major calorie sources is that they are easily controllable in a diet. Since the major sources are oils, you can very precisely titrate your "dose" by tablespoon and quite accurately substitute for other calorie sources without elaborate exchange guides.

Effects of Monounsaturated Fat–Carbohydrate Exchanges

- Stable or minimally increased or decreased total and LDL cholesterol levels
- Lowered total cholesterol/HDL ratio.
- Higher HDL cholesterol
- Higher HDL2 percentage
- Lower triglycerides
- Maintenance of subclass A status (if originally subclass A)

Other foods with relatively high "hidden" amounts of monos are: nuts, especially beechnuts, hickory nuts, walnuts; oat germ, salmon, lake trout, bluefish, capelin, carp, eel, Greenland halibut, king mackerel.

The Other Good Fats: Omega-3s

Ideally, about 1 to 2 percent of anybody's diet should consist of what are called the omega-3 fatty acids. ALA is a naturally occurring omega-3 found in vegetable products. Its more famous cousins, DHA and EPA, are the omega-3s found in fish oil, fish oil tablets, and other seafood. They are another major component of the Mediterranean diet, and they're responsible for the lower risk of Eskimo populations as well.

The makeup of fat in fish is quite different from that of land animals. Whereas the latter's fats are largely saturated, fish fats usually are about 30 percent mono and 40 percent polyunsaturated. Fish have saturated fats, too, but nothing like beef or poultry. In addition, they have the omega-3 fats:

Oil and Fat Content of Seafood

Omega-3 Content of 3½ oz (100 grams) Fish	Mgs. Omega-3	% Total Fat*
Anchovy	1,400	C
Bass, freshwater	300	B
Bass, striped	800	B
Bluefish	1,200	C
Carp	600	C
Catfish, Bullhead	500	D
Catfish, channel	300	C
Cod, Atlantic	300	A
Cod, Pacific	300	A
Eel	900	D
Flounder	200	A
Haddock	200	A
Halibut, Greenland	900	D
Halibut, Pacific	500	B
Herring, Atlantic	1,500	D
Herring, Pacific	900	D
Herring, round	1,300	D
Mackerel, Atlantic	2,600	D
Mackerel, chub	2,200	D

continues

Oil and Fat Content of Seafood *Continued*

Omega-3 Content of 3½ oz (100 grams) Fish	Mgs. Omega-3	% Total Fat*
Mackerel, horse	600	C
Mackerel, Japanese	1,900	D
Mackerel, king	2,200	B
Mullet	1,100	B
Ocean perch	200	B
Perch, white	400	A
Perch, yellow	300	A
Pike, northern	100	A
Pike, walleye	300	A
Pollock	500	A
Salmon, Atlantic	1,400	C
Salmon, chinook	1,500	D
Salmon, coho	1,000	C
Salmon, pink	1,000	C
Salmon, sockeye	1,300	D
Sea bass, Japanese	400	B
Shark	500	C
Sheepshard porgy	200	B
Smelt, pond	300	B
Smelt, rainbow	700	B
Smelt, sweet	300	B
Snapper, red	200	A
Sole, European	100	A
Swordfish	200	B
Trout, arctic char	600	B
Trout, brook	600	B
Trout, lake	2,000	D
Trout, rainbow	600	B
Tuna, albacore	600	A
Tuna, bluefin	1,600	C
Tuna, skipjack	400	A
Whitefish, lake	1,500	C
Whiting	100	A

Crustaceans (most not listed because of their high cholesterol content)

Crab, blue	400	B
Crab, Dungeness	300	A

Mollusks

Clam, soft-shell	400	A
Mussel, blue	500	B
Octopus	500	B
Oyster, Eastern	400	C

Omega-3 Content of 3½ oz (100 grams) Fish	Mgs. Omega-3	% Total Fat*
Oyster, European	500	B
Oyster, Pacific	600	B
Scallop	200	A
Squid, Atlantic	400	A

*A = 0–15% fat   B = 16–30% fat   C = 31–40% fat   D = >40% fat

For a 2,000-calorie diet, deriving 2 percent of fat from omega-3s means 40 calories or about 4½ grams—less than a fifth of an ounce! This means you could eat as much as three pounds per day of a low-fat fish like cod, or as little as six ounces of a very oily fish like mackerel. Though the recommendation of 1 percent to 2 percent of fat is ideal, for many people, especially those not living on the coasts, it may be impractical or too expensive.

In studies to determine just how much fish was needed to reduce risk for coronary artery disease, just ten ounces a week seemed enough. This should be in the form of real fish, because the so-called fish oil supplements actually contain high-calorie fats that you don't need. And there's another reason to eat real fish instead of supplements. The Physicians' Health Study compared men eating oily fish or lean fish like cod at least once a week, against men eating fish once a month. They found that those who ate fish more frequently, regardless of the fish, had half the rate of sudden cardiac death. The regular consumption of fish also substantially reduced risk for development or progression of coronary artery disease. The magnitude of this benefit is enormous: from 30 percent to 50 percent reduction in heart attacks. Furthermore, as the Physicians' Health Study indicated, the benefit is probably not limited to the omega-3 component of fish but also involves other mechanisms that are still not completely understood. So all fish seem to be beneficial, if eaten often enough.

We can include other forms of marine life in this category, most notably the mollusks, like clams and scallops. Though many crustaceans also provide omega-3 oils and are low in total fat, they also deliver a disproportionately high dose of cholesterol. Crustaceans such as shrimp and lobster should be avoided.

If weight loss is desirable, the highly beneficial effects of the oilier fish is blunted by their being higher in fat calories. So if your diet is to include daily or almost daily seafood, stick to the leaner varieties or much smaller portions of the fatty species. On the other hand, one or two high-fat fish per week won't do any damage to one's calorie counts while providing more than ample benefits.

A quick perusal of the list identifies king mackerel as delivering the biggest "bang for the buck," the least fat for the most omega-3s. Other fish with a high ratio of omega-3 to total fat are striped bass, Pacific halibut, mullet, pollock, rainbow smelts, trout, and the very common albacore tuna.

What exactly do the omega-3 fats do? The omega-3 molecule gets incorporated into the cell membrane of the endothelial cells, the immune and scavenger cells, and the platelets. These miraculous fatty acids protect the cell membranes from oxidation damage and can help inhibit everything from foam cell accumulation, to progressive fibrin deposition, to actual plaque rupture.

It's this last effect that has become most evident from the studies. You know that sudden cardiac death is usually caused by a sudden shutdown of a coronary artery. You also know this is the result of an atherosclerotic plaque rupturing and the blood clot created by that event. It makes perfect sense, then, that a substance that inhibits the ability of the platelets to start that clotting process would result in fewer deaths from cardiac arrest. Evidently it takes a very small amount of omega-3 fats to accomplish this—about 10 ounces of fish a week will do.

Larger doses of fish oils also help reduce the level of other risk factors for heart disease.

Omega-3 Effects on Risk Factors

- Reduces Triglyceride
- Reduces LDL Particles
- Reduces Apoprotein B
- Increases HDL Particles

Omega-3 fats in higher doses can also exert significant effects on circulating lipid-related risk factors. Reductions in triglyceride levels are their best known effects, but if you reduce the generation of LDL particles, then LDL cholesterol and Apoprotein B levels also fall. Additionally, HDL cholesterol levels will rise.

The mechanisms of these effects are not well understood. Nor is it worked out just which LDL particles are reduced and which HDL particles are raised. But the major impact on triglyc-

---

The Monounsaturated and Omega-3 Diet

- Fish daily or every other day
- Soybean products
- Beans
- Lentils
- Salads with olive and canola oil dressings

---

eride levels in itself indicates that the risk groups most benefiting from a diet high in omega-3 fat are similar to those benefiting from diets relatively high in monounsaturated fats.

Fortunately, many foods rich in omega-3s are also laden with monounsaturated fats. The most notable of these is canola oil, which, because of this, might actually have some advantages over olive oil.

Other Sources of Omega-3 Fats

Per 3½ ozs.	Omega-3	Total Fat (g)	Total Fat Calories
Soybeans, green and raw	3,200 mgs	7	63
Soybeans, mature seeds cooked	2,100 mgs	4.5	40
Soybeans, dried	1,600 mgs	2.1	190
Seaweed, spirilina (dried)	800 mgs	7.7	69
Leeks, raw	700 mgs	2.1	20
Navy beans	300 mgs	< 1	7
Pinto beans	300 mgs	< 1	8
Peas (dry)	200 mgs	2.4	22
Lima beans (dry)	200 mgs	1.4	13
Lentils (dry)	100 mgs	1.2	11
Cowpeas (dry)	300 mgs	2	18
Common bean (dry)	600 mgs	1.5	13
Canola oil	11,000 mgs	100	900
Soybean oil	6,800 mgs	100	900
Oat germ	1,400 mgs	30	270
Cod liver oil	25,500 mgs	100	900

Omega-3 Side Effects

As with everything else, moderation is important. A common problem found in Eskimo populations is a tendency to bleed. Because of their effects on platelet function and blood clotting, the benefits of eating a lot of fish can become a liability. This is especially important for people who have high blood pressure and, therefore, a higher risk for strokes caused by bleeding into the brain. It's also a factor for people with bleeding problems such as ulcers or inflammatory bowel conditions. So the same warnings that apply to taking aspirin are also relevant to consuming too much fish oil. Too much omega-3 can also depress the immune system and increase resistance to insulin in diabetics. So a balance must be struck: no more than 2 percent of your dietary calories should be omega-3s.

The Bad Fats: Omega-6 Polyunsaturated Fats

Not too many years ago, the omega-6 fats, more commonly referred to as the polyunsaturated fats, were heralded as the answer to high cholesterol, high-saturated-fat diets. Now we've become more sophisticated and have separated the three different kinds of polyunsaturated fats: omega-3s, natural omega-6s, and the "trans-fats."

Omega-6 fats are the naturally occurring fats found in vegetable oils. Taken in moderation, they provide a very beneficial component to the healthful diet. But because of their good publicity they've become an overemphasized component of many people's diets.

Discarding saturated fats for a diet rich in omega-6 polyunsaturated fats does result in impressive falls in LDL cholesterol levels. On average, the replacement of saturated with omega-6 fats for 1 percent of total dietary calories will lower total cholesterol by 1.4 mg. So replacing, say, 10 percent of calories from animal fats with vegetable oils yields a substantial decline in many people's total cholesterol level.

But there's a problem.

First, it's not just the LDL that falls. The HDL—especially HDL2—falls, too. This is okay if they fall in proportion, but in some people they don't. And second, the metabolism of omega-

Major Omega-6 Sources	
Safflower Oil	80%
Walnut Oil	70%
Sunflower Oil	70%
Corn Oil	62%
Soybean Oil	60%
Cottonseed Oil	62%
(Fish Oil	40%)

6 fats yields products that can predispose LDL particles to oxidation, thus making them tend to produce atherosclerosis while reducing their overall cholesterol content.

These become very real concerns when omega-6 fats constitute more than 10 percent of the diet—a very common problem with many "heart-healthy" diets.

Changing meal preparation habits can substantially reduce the omega-6s in the diet. Using olive oil or canola oil for salad dressings and in cooking is one step in the right direction. Limiting the intake of "low-cholesterol" and "low-saturated-fat" commercially produced food items is another. Almost all of the fat in these products is either omega-6 polyunsaturated fats or our last group of problem fats, the "trans-fats."

The Ugly Fats: Trans-Fats

While polyunsaturated omega-6 fats have some problems because they've been overused, the trans-fats are truly ugly creatures. These are not natural fats at all but are polyunsaturated fats that have been deformed by human manipulation. The resulting Frankenstein has become a public health problem.

The food manufacturing industry decided to transform polyunsaturated vegetable fats, which are liquid at room temperature, into tantalizing butterlike solids. So they added hydrogens to the molecule's carbon chains to make them solid at room temperature—more like butter. Thus, the promise of the best of both worlds: the health benefits of vegetable oils with the irresistible look, feel, and taste of animal fat.

So what's the problem? Thinking the transformation was okay because it involved a fat that was originally polyunsaturated proved extremely naive. When trans-fats are incorporated into the structure of the LDL particle they make that particle highly disposed to oxidation. They will also increase the numbers of particles and one's LDL cholesterol levels, as fully saturated fats do—though not as much. To compound that problem, HDL and especially HDL2 levels fall, and there's some evidence that even Lp(a) levels can rise. These are, indeed, ugly effects.

Effects of Trans-Fats on Risk Factors

- Increase LDL Cholesterol
- Increase Apo B
- Decrease HDL Cholesterol
- Decrease HDL2
- Questionably Increase Lp(a)
- LDL Oxidation
- Increase Total Cholesterol / HDL Ratio

Where do you find them? Look for the term "hydrogenated or partially hydrogenated vegetable oil." These will be found in a vast array of commercially prepared foods.

Trans-Fat Sources

Butter

Milk fat

Animal fats

Fried foods: meats, fish, chicken, vegetables

Commercially baked goods: cookies, cakes, pies, crackers

Margarine

High-fat snacks: potato chips, corn chips, tortilla chips

Other snacks

A few years ago, the results of a number of studies signaling the trans-fat problem caused a swing back to the use of "natural" fats for eating and cooking. People switched back from margarine to butter. But as bad as margarine may be, it's still only about 10 percent saturated plus 1 percent trans, while butter is 60 percent saturated and 5 percent trans! There's really no contest here. Margarine is still better than butter, the softer tub margarine being the best. But *both* are bad. As a basic rule, if fat is solid at room temperature, it's bad for you. Trans-fats, which constitute about 4 to 5 percent of the typical American diet, should be grouped together with saturated fats; the two combined should not constitute more than 6 percent of your diet's calories.

Saturated Fat Hit List

Palm-Kernel Oil	81% sat. fat
Coconut Oil	92% sat. fat
Palm Oil	51% sat. fat
Butter	66% sat. fat
Cocoa Butter	63% sat. fat

Saturated Fats

These go by the names lauric, myristic, and palmitic acid. Palmitic is the biggest culprit in the American diet, providing 60 percent of the saturated fat in the average diet. It is mostly found in animal foods. The other two fats though, are more sinister—they pose as vegetarian health foods, but they are among the most lethal things that grow in the ground. Their aliases are palm-kernel oil, coconut oil, and palm oil. Watch for them in product labels. Like trans-fats, they are ubiquitous.

Fiber

No discussion of diet can be complete without mentioning fiber. The proper fiber intake can preclude the use of medications if the diet guidelines we've already cited are followed and fail to achieve the desired ends.

Fiber primarily reduces LDL cholesterol levels. It does this by a number of mechanisms. Perhaps most important, it binds with cholesterol in the intestinal tract to prevent absorption. This is identical to the mechanism of certain of the anticholesterol drugs. The fiber that's been shown to so effectively do this is called beta-glucan, found in oat bran.

It seems the higher one's cholesterol is to start with, the more pronounced the effect. The average LDL cholesterol level reduction one can expect is around 15 percent, the effect sometimes being evident in less than a month and certainly after two to four months of a high-fiber diet.

Studies using fiber of various sorts also show mild elevations of HDL and lowering of triglycerides. For diabetics and insulin-resistant people who aren't overtly diabetic, improvement in blood sugar insulin responses have also been demonstrated.

There are two kinds of fiber. Soluble fiber is the fiber that binds cholesterol. Insoluble fiber doesn't affect risk levels per se. But it has other very compelling benefits, such as being an aid in weight loss and digestion and decreasing transit time of food in the bowel, which therefore minimizes absorption of full caloric loads and exposure to toxic contaminants.

The generic term "fiber" as used in product labels means the combination of both kinds of fibers. For reduction of cholesterol levels one needs at least 3 to 6 grams of soluble fiber daily. Different forms of fiber will contain different ratios of soluble to insoluble fiber, so you must be careful to understand just what it is you're eating.

Amounts of Various Foods Delivering 1 Gram of Soluble Fiber

Food	Amount	Total Fiber Delivered (Grams)
Fruits		
apple, unpeeled	2½ (2¾″) whole	8
apple, peeled	5 (2¾″) whole	10
applesauce	1½ cups	4.5
apricot	5 halves	3.5
apricot, dried	12 halves	3
avocado	½ whole	4

Food	Amount	Total Fiber Delivered (Grams)
banana	16 (8″)	7
blackberries	1¼ cups	12.3
blueberries	2½ cups	10.5
cantaloupe	5 cups cubed	3
cherries, canned	3 cups	4
cranberry sauce	3½	3.5
dates	30 whole	43
figs	6 whole	10
fruit cocktail	3½ cups	4.5
grapefruit, whole	1 (5″ diam.)	4
grapefruit, without membrane	3½ (5″ diam.)	4
honeydew melon	5 cups cubed	5
kiwifruit	3 medium	4.5
nectarine	3 (2½″ diam.)	2.5
orange	2 (2½″) whole	4.5
papaya	5 cups cubed	15
peach, peeled	4 (2½″)	2.5
peach, unpeeled	4 (2½″)	3.5
pear, canned	6 halves	5
pear, unpeeled	1½ medium	5
pineapple	5 cups cubed	7
plum	6 medium size	2.5
plum, canned	7½ medium size	3
prune, dried	5 whole	3
prune, fresh	10 medium size	5
raisins	1¼ cups	8
raspberries	1½ cups	8
rhubarb	2½ cups	5.5
strawberries	1½ cups	4
tangerine	10 (2½″)	15
Vegetables		
artichoke	¼ of 1 medium	1.5
asparagus	18 spears	5
bamboo shoots	5 cups slices	1
beans, green or yellow wax	1½ cups	4.5
beet	1 cup	3
beet greens	1½ cups	5
bok choy	5 cups shredded	12
broccoli	10 stalks	9
brussels sprouts	1¼ cups	8
cabbage, green, cooked	5 cups shredded	17
carrot	1¼ cups slices	4
cauliflower	2½ cups pieces	6
celery	30 stalks (5″)	11
collards	2½ cups chopped	14.5

continues

159

Amounts of Various Foods Delivering 1 Gram of Soluble Fiber *Continued*

Food	Amount	Total Fiber Delivered (Grams)
Vegetables *Continued*		
corn, creamed	1½ cups	4
corn, whole kernel	5 cups	16
corn, on cob	10 ears (3½″ diam.)	10
eggplant	2½ cups sliced	6
kali	1½ cups chopped	7.5
kohlrabi	2½ cups sliced	8
mushroom	20 medium	3
mushroom, canned	2½ cups	10
mustard greens	2½ cups	11
okra	1 cup	3.3
onion	5 cups chopped	12
parsnip	1 cup chopped	5
pea pods	2½	9
pepper, green or chili	5 cups chopped	9
potato, red, peeled	5 (2½″ diam.)	3
potato, red, unpeeled	3 (2½″ diam.)	4
potato, white, peeled	5 (2½″ diam.)	5
potato, white, unpeeled	1 (2½″ diam.)	4
pumpkin	¾ cup	5.5
rutabaga	1½ cups cubes	5.5
spinach, canned or cooked	1½ cups	7
spinach, raw	6 cups	7
squash, acorn, butternut	1½ cups cubed	5.5
squash, yellow	5½ cups slices	7
sweet potato	2 (5″ × 2″)	4
tomato	5 medium	4
Grain Products		
biscuit	20 (2″ × 1″)	5
bread, French	2½ slices	4
bread, Italian	5 slices	4
bread, raisin	5 slices	3.5
bread, rye	5 slices	3.5
bread, whole wheat	3 slices	7.5
cereal, All Bran	½ cup	12
cereal, 40% Bran Flakes	½ cup	9
cereal, cooked, oatmeal	½ cup	1.8
(Quaker Oat and other brands)		
cereal, corn flakes	10 cups	12
cereal, Cream of Wheat	2½ cups	4.5
cereal, Frosted Mini Wheat	20 biscuits	12.5
cereal, Golden Grahams	10 cups	8

Food	Amount	Total Fiber Delivered (Grams)
cereal, Granola	¾ cup	4
cereal, Grapenut	2½ cups	6.5
cereal, Grapenuts	¾ cup	5
cereal, Life	1 cup	3
cereal, Oat Bran	½ cup	2.5
cereal, Product 19	10 cups	19
cereal, Puffed Wheat	3 cups	2.7
cereal, Rice Krispies	10 cups	5
cereal, Shredded Wheat	3 pieces	8
cereal, Smacks	5 cups	3.5
cereal, Special K	10 cups	7
cereal, Wheat Chex	1½ cups	5
cereal, Wheaties	2 cups	6
cookie, fig	3 oz.	3.5
cookie, oatmeal	3 oz.	2.7
corn bread	10 (2½″ × 2½″ pieces)	14
flour, white or wheat	10 tbsp.	2
muffin, commercial	5 oz.	9
muffin, English	3	5
muffin, wheat bran	4 oz.	7
noodles, chow mein	2½ cups	4
pancake, buckwheat	6 (4″ cake)	8
pasta	2½ cups	5
stuffing, cornbread	2½ cups	5.5
wheat germ	¾ cup	12
Legumes		
baked beans, canned	¼ cup	2.75
beans, black, cooked	2½ cups	14
beans, great northern, cooked	1½ cups	25
beans, kidney, canned	½ cup	4.5
beans, lima, cooked	2 cups	7
beans, navy, cooked	2½ cups	15.5
beans, pigeon	2½ cups	18.5
lentils, cooked	2½ cups	14.5
peas, black-eyed, cooked	2½ cups	14
peas, green, canned	1½ cups	19
pea soup	1¼ cups	3.75
Nuts and Seeds		
almonds	10 oz.	25
cashews	10 oz.	13
peanut	10 oz.	19
peanut butter	10 oz.	16
pecans	10 oz.	17
Supplements		
psyllium (Metamucil)	⅓ tsp.	1.3

Because different foods have different ratios of soluble to insoluble fiber, I've included a fairly extensive list of the fiber contents of foods commonly used as fiber sources. As you can see, the variation in relative fiber content is *very* wide, and the desired amount of "fiber foods" is enormous when compared to the typical American diet. There are many foods high in insoluble fiber that if relied upon as your principal sources of *soluble* fiber will give you a lot of bathroom time. One of the most convenient ways to take care of one's soluble fiber requirement is by taking one or two teaspoons of Metamucil daily.

Regardless of your method, eating enough fiber may require a gradual buildup of tolerance to the laxative and cramping effects many people get with even slightly increased intakes of fruits and cereals.

Every diet should contain an adequate selection of high-fiber foods to ensure a daily intake of 3 to 6 grams of soluble fiber, and 25 to 30 grams total fiber.

Putting It All Together

If your risk profile indicates you need a low-fat, high-carbohydrate diet, you should begin with a 30 percent fat diet. After six weeks if the improvement in LDL levels is not satisfactory, push the fat percentage down to 25 or 20 percent. If at these levels triglycerides shoot up more than 100 percent to beyond 200, and certainly if above 400, your HDL, LDL subclass, and possibly your HDL subclass should be rechecked. At least check your total cholesterol to HDL ratio. It shouldn't rise.

Subclass B people with low triglycerides can start at the 25 to 20 percent fat level, as they are less likely to see these steep rises.

People who require "normal" fat diets should follow the 40 percent outline. How much fat is 40 percent? Or 30 percent, or 20 percent for that matter? There's a very simple way to figure this out.

The following table matches body weight to daily caloric needs for sedentary and moderately active people. Moderately active means you have a job or do housework that keeps you on your feet and moving most of the day. (Active exercisers need more calories, and that is discussed in chapter 14.)

Daily Caloric Intake

	Sedentary	
Weight	*Men*	*Women*
100	1,500	1,300
120	1,800	1,550
140	2,100	1,800
160	2,400	2,100
180	2,700	2,350
200	3,000	2,400
220	3,300	2,660

	Moderately Active	
Weight	*Men*	*Women*
100	2,100	1,800
120	2,500	2,150
140	2,950	2,500
160	3,250	2,880
180	3,780	3,250
200	4,200	3,600
220	4,600	3,650

Regardless of which category of the overall fat percentage diet you fall in, the following rules should be used in structuring your initial selections of foods:

- minimum of one to two fish meals (any fish) per week
- trans-fats and saturated fats less than 7% of total calories
- cholesterol less than 150 mg day (< 300 mg for Apoprotein E 3/2)
- sugar less than 10% of calories (see exceptions in chapter 14)
- polyunsaturated fats less than 10% of calories
- monounsaturated fats: 25 to 30% of calories (40% fat diet); 15–20% of calories (30% fat diet); 10–15% of calories (25% fat diet)

How Much Fat in a Low-Fat Diet?

$$40\% \text{ fat diet} = \frac{\text{calories} \times .4}{9} = \text{grams fat per day}$$

$$30\% \text{ fat diet} = \frac{\text{calories} \times .3}{9} = \text{grams fat per day}$$

$$20\% \text{ fat diet} = \frac{\text{calories} \times .2}{9} = \text{grams fat per day}$$

Bad Fats: What's Your Limit?

$$\text{grams saturated fat permitted per day} = \frac{\text{calories} \times .07}{9}$$

$$\text{example:} \quad 2,000 \text{ calorie diet} = \frac{2,000 \times .07}{9} = 16 \text{ grams saturated fat}$$

Good Fats: What's Your Limit?

$$\text{monounsaturated fats: } 40\% \text{ fat diet} \frac{\text{calories} \times .3}{9} = \text{grams monounsaturated fat}$$

$$30\% \text{ fat diet} \frac{\text{calories} \times .2}{9} = \text{grams monounsaturated fat}$$

$$20\% \text{ fat diet} \frac{\text{calories} \times .15}{9} = \text{grams monounsaturated fat}$$

If your system cannot tolerate low fats then increase monoun-saturated fats by 9 calories (1 gram) for every 12 calories (3 grams) of carbohydrate being replaced.

How Low Can You Go?

This is the other side of the coin. Those who respond to a low-fat diet—subclass B people who are Apoprotein 4/3 and 4/4, and some 3/3s; and the subclass As who are Apoprotein E4s—will see dramatic responses in LDL levels. The subclass Bs are also much more likely to see corresponding decreases in their Apoprotein B levels which indicates not only that the LDL cholesterol content of their LDL particles is falling but so are the numbers of particles.

If this happens, and there are no adverse effects on HDL and total cholesterol/HDL ratio, there's no reason not to push further, especially if LDL levels still remain high or you have one of these reasons for driving your LDL level as low as possible:

- Active coronary artery disease
- Positive family history of premature coronary artery disease
- No family history but more than two major risk factors
- Other genetic risk factors resistant to control

If LDL levels are over 100, triglycerides are not skyrocketing, your LDL subclass status is stable, and HDL levels are stable and in proportion to LDL levels, then you may benefit from dropping from a 30 percent to a 20 percent fat diet. If 20 percent fat diet is tolerated, further benefits in this group of responsive people may be enjoyed at 15 percent and even 10 percent fat levels. There are many people who tolerate a 10 percent fat diet quite well. The keys are your genetic predispositions and keeping your intake of *simple* carbohydrates minimal—below 10 percent or even 5 percent of calories.

Alcohol

There is some evidence that beer, wine, and spirits each have beneficial effects against heart disease. Alcohol seems to raise HDL, but it's mostly HDL3. There are other substances in both beer and red wine that exert other protective effects as well. One glass of wine or beer or an ounce of whiskey a day probably won't hurt you. But alcohol is also a very potent elevator of triglycerides. If triglycerides are a problem, alcohol should be severely restricted. And in any case, a drink a day is not a substitute for exercise, a good diet, or necessary medication. Unfortunately, some people think it is.

What Diet Won't Do for You

There is very little evidence that the proper diet can convert an LDL subclass B distribution to the much lower risk subclass A state. This observation brings us to one of the as yet unresolved issues about the independence of the subclass B state as a risk factor.

Many non–North American population groups who exist on diets composed almost exclusively of unrefined, complex carbohydrates, and nonanimal or marine animal sources of protein and fat have high percentages of LDL subclass B people, yet they also have low rates of coronary artery disease. Obviously, there's more to atherosclerosis than we now know.

A diet high in complex carbohydrates and low in saturated fat with primarily seafood as the source of protein and fat robs the atherosclerosis process of its raw molecular materials. This is not completely evident in the tests available to us, but it is probably why these large population groups can exist quite nicely in the subclass B state.

The subclass B individual who radically restructures his or her diet in the ways I've outlined to reach goal risk factor levels for LDL, Apoprotein B, and HDL is much better off despite not having converted to subclass A. The parallel risk model maintains that this person *still* remains theoretically at high risk by virtue of the subclass state; but now we enter a gray area of knowledge. Is he really? Or have the dangers been taken out of the subclass B particles and the toxic stew that usually surrounds them? There are strong opinions about these questions, but few solid answers.

Diet is only one part of the three-part behavioral modification program that *every* person at risk for heart disease must adopt. So, to an important degree, the question is moot. The high-risk person will rarely convert his or her risk profile to goal levels on the basis of diet alone. Proper weight maintenance and exercise are almost always needed to complete the picture. It is through these two areas that changes in LDL particle size and subclass status can be achieved. Only after that has failed do we confront the issue of whether an asymptomatic person, who may also be young, who is at appropriate body mass index (see page 168), is on the proper diet, and does enough exercise, should go on a lifetime of medications because of resistant subclass B status.

13

Step Eight:
Lose Weight Now

For many people, the key to minimizing or even eliminating their heart disease risks is attaining the proper weight. But proper weight is not to be taken for granted. Your risk factor profile will determine the right weight for you. And how your weight is distributed may be a clue to your risk factor profile.

Risk Factors Minimized by Weight Loss

small LDL particle size
high LDL cholesterol levels
LDL subclass B
increased Apoprotein B
low HDL cholesterol
low HDL2
high triglycerides
reduced insulin sensitivity
diabetes
high blood pressure
high fibrinogen levels
depressed intrinsic fibrinolysis

What's Your Appropriate Weight?

Don't go to a standard height-weight chart. Hidden within the normal range of weights for your height can be an appreciable amount of excess body fat devouring precious HDLs and churning out triglycerides to poison the LDL particles. Instead, you should use body mass index, or BMI.

Body Mass Index

Your body mass index is more than a measure of appropriate weight for height. It is a calculation of your body's composition and reflects the appropriate level of fat for your size and shape.

Your Body Mass Index

Height	Body Weight in Pounds													
4'10"	91	95	100	105	110	115	119	124	129	134	138	143	167	191
4'11"	94	99	104	109	114	119	124	128	133	138	143	148	173	198
5'	97	102	107	112	118	123	128	133	138	143	148	153	179	204
5'1"	100	106	111	116	122	127	132	137	143	148	153	158	185	211
5'2"	104	109	115	120	126	131	136	142	147	153	158	164	191	218
5'3"	107	113	118	124	130	135	141	146	152	158	163	169	197	225
5'4"	110	116	122	128	134	140	145	151	157	163	169	174	203	232
5'5"	114	120	126	132	138	144	150	156	162	168	174	180	210	240
5'6"	118	124	130	136	142	148	155	161	167	173	179	186	216	247
5'7"	121	127	134	140	146	153	159	166	172	178	185	191	223	255
5'8"	125	131	138	144	151	158	164	171	177	184	190	197	230	262
5'9"	128	135	142	149	155	162	169	176	182	189	196	203	236	270
5'10"	132	139	146	153	160	167	174	181	188	195	202	207	243	278
5'11"	136	143	150	157	165	172	179	186	193	200	208	215	250	286
6'	140	147	154	162	169	177	184	191	199	206	213	221	258	294
6'1"	144	151	159	166	174	182	189	197	204	212	219	227	265	302
6'2"	148	155	163	171	179	186	194	202	210	218	225	233	272	311
6'3"	152	160	168	176	184	192	200	208	216	224	232	240	279	319
6'4"	156	164	172	180	189	197	205	213	221	230	238	246	287	328
BMI	*19*	*20*	*21*	*22*	*23*	*24*	*25*	*26*	*27*	*28*	*29*	*30*	*35*	*40*

To determine your BMI, just find your correct height on the left column and move horizontally to find your weight. The number at the bottom of the selected weight column is the BMI. You're at the right weight if your BMI is between 20 and 25. Traditionally, you are considered overweight if your BMI is greater than 25, and "obesity" officially starts at a BMI of 30. Above 35 and you have a serious medical problem. However, for many people, BMIs in the high "normal" range of 24 to 25 are still too high. In fact, recent studies have forced a downward revision of acceptable BMI, and many people, as you will see, are actually unacceptably overweight, even though they fall within the "normal" BMI ranges as indicated in standard charts.

High BMI by itself represents a cardiovascular risk factor, but the mechanisms by which excess fat increases risk are complex and involve almost all of the other risk factors listed at the beginning of this chapter. In the traditional studies, mortality rates begin to rise above the BMI 25 point. They also rise below the 20 point, so being too skinny is not the answer either.

A 10 percent gain in body weight increases your risk for heart attack by about 25 percent. A woman with a BMI of 29, for example, raises her risks more than 200 percent compared to someone in the lower end of the normal range.

BMI can be misleading when dealing with extremely muscular athletes like bodybuilders. NFL linemen have BMIs in the 35 to 39 range, while relatively less muscular basketball players are just above normal at 26. There are compendiums of normal ranges for these "abnormal" situations so that even within these groups the athletes with excess fat can be detected. But unless you're all bulked up, normal ranges apply.

There is a lot of latitude within the range of normal BMI. A person six feet tall, for example, should weigh between 147 and 184 to have a normal BMI. That's a big range—almost forty pounds—and that forty pounds can hide a lot of risk factors. So just being in the normal BMI range may not be sufficient to decrease your risk. You have to be a little more precise, and there are two ways to do this.

The first method requires no more equipment than a tape measure and reference to Figure 5: Figure out your waist-hip ratio. This information can sharpen the resolution of the BMI reading you take off the chart because it tells you something about the distribution of your extra weight. To get your waist-hip ratio just measure your waist and hips at the widest point.

Then using a ruler or the side of a sheet of paper, line up your two readings. The point where the ruler crosses the center line is your waist-hip ratio. For women, it should be smaller than .8, and men smaller than 1. An elevated ratio means you have too much abdominal fat, the kind of fat that actively sequesters triglycerides, mostly from eating excess carbohydrates. In a sense, that fat gobbles up HDLs as well. This excess fat creates another problem: It makes insulin levels rise, and this promotes the production of even more triglycerides. These triglycerides become packaged in the VLDL particles that eventually become small dense LDL particles.

169

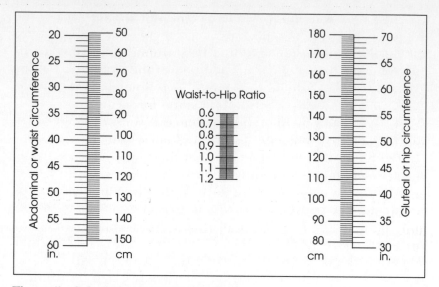

Figure 5. Calculating Waist-to-Hip Ratio

It's not surprising then that there is a very strong correlation with LDL subclass B, high triglyceride levels, high LDL levels, low HDL and HDL2 levels on the one hand, and elevated waist-hip ratios on the other. It's quite possible to be overweight and to have a high BMI with a normal waist-hip ratio. It's also quite possible to be overweight and be LDL subclass A. The added information the waist hip-ratio conveys is to give some indication of the nature of the underlying metabolic processes that lead to increased risk.

Women have a lower waist-hip ratio because it's normal for them to concentrate fat in their thighs and buttocks. That's because estrogen operates *below* the belt to stimulate the enzymes that cause the fat accumulation. For reasons not well understood, this distribution of fat in women is much more benign. After menopause, this reverses, and women at high risk for diabetes and for conversion to subclass B can gain a lot of abdominal fat just as men do. (When this occurs, it's an indication for estrogen therapy.)

If you know you have a normal BMI and an elevated waist-to-hip ratio, your proper point on the BMI range should be closer to 21 than 25. You'll know when you've reached that point when you convert your waist-hip ratio to where it should be and/or when your risk profile improves.

You can also do this the other way around: Check your risk profile, then your BMI. If you have few of the risk factors listed earlier, then your BMI is appropriate. This is no guarantee you'll like the way you look, but you are at the medically appropriate weight. Not all normal BMIs are the same. A study of 62,000 men and 262,000 women (the American Cancer Society's gigantic Cancer Prevention Study) found that the higher range of BMI may indeed mask significant risk factors in that excess fat. In all but the oldest age groups, the BMIs in the "high normal" range as measured by traditional standards carried significantly higher mortality statistics from both all causes and from heart disease alone.

Optimal BMI According to Age

Men	
Age	*Optimal Range of BMI*
30–44	21–22
45–54	21–22
55–64	21–23
65–74	21–26

Women	
Age	*Optimal Range of BMI*
30–44	21–23
45–54	21–22
55–64	21–24
65–74	21–28

As you can see, what has been traditionally considered the normal range of BMI is no longer believed to be optimal for most age groups. In fact, people who are above the newly revised optimal ranges increase their likelihood for coronary artery disease by at least 20 percent just on the basis of the added fat weight. This, of course, is not true for everyone—the waist-hip ratio being a very helpful indicator of who should pay particular attention to these new guidelines.

The story gets worse at higher levels of excess fat. Listed below are the BMI levels at or above which each group increases their statistical risk by 50 percent.

Men		Women	
Age	*BMI*	*Age*	*BMI*
30–44	25	30–44	27
45–54	26	45–54	26
55–64	28	55–64	30
65–74	33	65–74	32

So if you have a normal BMI with an elevated waist-hip ratio, check your lipid profile. If any of the listed factors are elevated, choose as your goal a weight nearer the lower limit of the BMI range. As a starting point, use the values listed above to select the target weight. For example, low HDL with a BMI of 25. Age fifty male. Find the weight at BMI 23 on the BMI chart and subtract from your present weight. If already at that weight, go to next lower BMI point.

Your Best Weight

There are only two ways to lose weight, and they have to be done together: exercise and reduce calories. It is a simple equation: calories *in* must be less than calories *out*. There are no magic formulas, diets, potions, or pills that change that basic thermodynamic law. It is an immutable law of physics.

In the previous chapter, you learned approximately how many calories you need to eat each day. The proper weight loss should be no more than two pounds a week. If you lose more than that, then you lose muscle. As you'll learn in the next chapter, muscle is the most potent natural weapon your body has to change risk factors.

Losing a pound of fat requires eating 3,500 fewer calories a week, or 500 fewer calories a day. If you've been at your present weight for a long time, you are in a metabolic equilibrium where your appetite equals your needs. Within the range of normal BMI, it is often very difficult to shed more than a few pounds.

This is your "set point," the preferred weight your body maintains without conscious intervention on your part, and budging beyond it is very difficult. There's a multibillion-dollar industry built upon this phenomenon: You pay a weight-loss program money to use their magic diet plan and you lose ten or twenty pounds beyond your set point. Then you bounce right back to your original weight, and sign up for another expensive program to lose the same ten or twenty pounds. Repeat customers are good business.

Losing weight within your BMI range—assuming you are at your consistently stable weight—requires two changes: daily, or almost daily, increase of caloric expenditure with no increase in caloric intake, and a change in the composition, but not necessarily the number, of calories of your diet.

Of course, this means daily exercise. A 500-calorie energy expenditure is five miles of running. A very fit person can do that in less than an hour on a treadmill or NordicTrack. Using exercise alone to lose weight usually does not work. That's because exercisers will use their workouts as a signal to overeat. You must keep your calories constant while continuing to exercise.

The other half of this problem is restructuring your diet. This is the complicated part, because the best diet for you will depend on your Apoprotein E and LDL subclass status; otherwise it might be opposing the effects of weight loss.

"Normal" fat diets should be structured so that the major carbohydrate intake comes shortly after the exercise period, as well as *during* the exercise period when engaged in endurance work. You train muscles to burn fat by *exercise*, not diet. You eat carbohydrate in the postexercise period to replenish muscle stores of high energy sugar.

The absolutely crucial aspect of this regimen is that you count your calories in the beginning and make sure there's *no* increase in eating as a result of exercise.

For people who require low-fat diets, the same principles apply with the added warning to eliminate sugary foods like the ones listed in chapter 12. With one exception, they must be replaced with fiber-rich, complex-carbohydrate sources. This will eliminate the wild insulin swings so many people on "low-fat" diets experience. Insulin promotes deposition of fat in that abdominal fat region. The exception is just before, during, and in the four hours following exercise. At these times sugary snacks, fruit drinks, and low-fat candies go straight to your muscles, where you need the sugar.

Supplementing aerobic exercise with resistance training can also be useful. A half hour three times a week on Nautilus machines or lifting weights will stimulate muscle building and greatly contribute to the fat loss. The reshaping of the body is the key. In fact, you might not even notice that much change in your weight. What should be changing is the waist-to-hip ratio. That is the much more sensitive indicator of *fat* weight loss. It is this measurement, not your weight, that will signal where your proper place in the BMI range is.

For people above their normal BMI range, exercise won't be enough, and caloric restriction must be planned. Your initial target weight should be one that places you in the upper range of your normal BMI. Don't be too ambitious.

The weight loss should be planned so that no more than two pounds of fat per week are lost. That means a caloric deficit of about 1,000 calories a day in a combination of reduced eating and daily or almost daily exercise. On rest days, eat less. People with BMIs greater than 30 need professional help for their weight loss. Such people must consult a dietitian or nutritionist, and may require medical help as well.

Effects of Weight Loss on Risk Factors

Weight loss raises HDL and lowers triglycerides. If fat weight loss is accomplished by holding calories constant and exercising, HDL cholesterol and HDL2 percentages will rise appreciably. Rise of HDL cholesterol by as much as 50 percent can be expected. If a low-fat diet had been adopted at the same time, the exercise effect will maintain HDL and HDL2 levels that might otherwise fall with the lower fat intake.

Triglycerides can be expected to plummet. Exercise and the fat weight loss will oppose the tendency in subclass B people to raise triglycerides in response to a high-carbohydrate diet.

Another response to weight loss will be that LDL particle size will shift to larger, less dense particles. In addition, LDL cholesterol levels will fall. The net fall will be the result of a complex interaction among your LDL subclass, Apoprotein E type, the composition of your diet, and the amount of fat weight lost. The decline in LDL level is impossible to predict with accuracy.

Finally, reduction of excess fat can improve insulin sensitivity to the extent that some diabetics don't need insulin or medicine. This improved sensitivity will also benefit your lipid risk-factor profile.

In this chapter, I have concentrated on people who may think that their weight is normal. Your waist-hip ratio and circulating risk factor profile are intimately linked to the presence of excess fat. But just as with those who have "normal" cholesterol levels, those whose body weight is normal may have a body composition so unbalanced that risk is as high as for those who are obese. The next chapter will show you exactly what you must do to retrain your metabolism to keep fat weight off.

14

Step Nine:
Get on an
Exercise Program Now

Aerobic exercise is crucial. Whether we're talking about metabolism, physiology, the clotting of the blood, or the form foods take when they are absorbed into the body, exercise has to enter into the discussion. Practically every cardiac risk factor can be countered by exercise, and the more exercise is scientifically examined, the more profound its effects are found to be. We are coming to appreciate that exercise is not just an essential behavioral contribution to longevity; it is the most essential.

Many studies demonstrate the unquestionable benefits of exercise. These studies clearly show that in a large population, exercise reduces overall rates of heart disease and heart attack. They also define certain levels of exercise necessary to achieve any benefit. But like any large epidemiological study, they say nothing about the individual's response. You can't tell from population studies what specific benefit exercise may hold for you.

In the early 1990s, a report on the long-term effects of exercise on over 10,000 Harvard alumni reconfirmed its importance in the control of disease. First, it showed very clearly that there was a close relationship between the amount of physical exercise, longevity, and the risk for heart disease. In this study, the people expending as few as 500 calories a week in exercise enjoyed modest improvements in risk, whereas those expending 2,000 calories a week (the equivalent of twenty miles of running at four miles per hour) enjoyed very significant reductions in heart disease risk. This benefit was dose dependent up to a level of 3,500 calories a week (thirty-five miles of running), then it leveled off. The people exercising the most had about half as much risk of coronary artery disease as those exercising least.

This report also showed that nobody who exercised below a certain level of intensity benefited from the exercise. That intensity level was about 300 to 400 calories per hour, or a walk or run at a pace of three to four miles per hour.

Studies performed on Norwegian and Finnish men also found that those who exercised the most reaped the greatest benefits. In addition, these studies also found a threshold effect. When it is surpassed, it yields a big jump in benefit. A Finnish study of over 1,400 men, for instance, demonstrated a jump from marginal levels of protection against developing coronary artery disease to a breathtaking 55 percent reduction when the exercise intensity reached a level of over 600 calories an hour or a running pace of six miles per hour. Combining this level of intensity with long duration amplified the protective benefit.

The studies show that for the population as a whole, there is an incontestable linear relationship between fitness and protection from coronary artery disease. It has been calculated that for every hour you exercise, you add two hours to your life span. But achieving this benefit requires a knowledge of your own risk factors. The kind and amount of exercise that is best for you depends on your profile of risks, which is a profile different from anyone else's.

There are three dimensions to exercise: intensity, duration, and frequency. Intensity describes how much energy you expend in a given period of time, duration is how long you exercise, and frequency is how often. Depending on your risk factors, you need a different balance of these three dimensions.

Exercise benefits people in two distinct ways. First, there are muscular, or mechanical, benefits. Exercise changes the size and density of muscles—all muscles, including the heart. Exercising to the point of muscle fiber exhaustion or overload of the muscle causes it to become thicker and denser so that the next time the same load won't fatigue it. For this kind of mechanical benefit, higher intensity, shorter duration, and less frequency are optimal.

And second, exercise changes the metabolic state of the body—it changes how the muscles process fuel, which in turn changes the chemistry of the blood. This change in the blood chemistry is one of the things that protects you from a heart attack: The changes affect almost all of the circulating risk factors for cardiovascular disease. For this kind of metabolic benefit, lower intensity, longer duration, and increased frequency are essential.

Mechanical Benefits of Exercise

Higher intensity exercise causes the heart to become physically stronger. As the heart muscle grows, the network of blood vessels enriching this increased mass becomes richer and more complex. Blood flow through the athletic heart is richer and faster. Where there is a partial blockage of a coronary artery (the arteries that feed the heart), the athletically fit heart is better at pumping blood through that smaller passageway. The athletic heart's muscle fibers contract much more efficiently. This means much more power can be generated for any given blood flow level, and the margins of safety are expanded. In addition, exercise gives the heart anatomic flexibility to impaired blood flow. The blood vessels supplying the muscle have expanded and branched off, even forming conduits around the area of the original artery's blockage, entirely circumventing the problem of limited flow. All of this follows from strengthening the heart muscle.

The Mechanical Benefits of Exercise

- Increased efficiency of ventricular contraction
- Decreased heart rate at rest and for every level of exercise
- Decreased blood pressure
- Decreased overall work of heart at rest
- Decreased stimulatory (adrenalinelike) hormone levels
- Increased volume of blood pumped for any level of energy used by heart muscle
- Decreased resistance to blood flow in the circulation
- Reduced susceptibility of heart to irregular heart rhythms
- Rerouting of blood flow from blocked and partially blocked coronary arteries into alternative vessels
- Proliferation of small blood vessels supplying heart muscle
- Remodeling of partially blocked coronaries to minimize level of blood flow being blocked by existing plaques

In the same way it conditions the arteries of the heart, exercise also conditions the arteries of the rest of the body and their end points, the capillaries that feed the exercising muscles. For any given amount of blood pumped, a circulation conditioned by exercise allows the heart to move it with less resistance; the heart's contraction needs to generate less force. And because less force is needed, less coronary blood flow is needed to supply the contracting heart muscles. The entire system becomes more efficient and more resistant to the effects atherosclerosis can have on limiting blood flow.

Metabolic Benefits of Exercise

Exercise not only strengthens muscles but also changes the chemistry of the blood.

The Metabolic Benefits of Exercise

- Increases LDL particle size
- Shifts the particle distribution from the subclass B range toward subclass A
- Lowers LDL cholesterol levels
- Lowers triglyceride levels
- Raises HDL and HDL2 levels
- Lowers insulin levels
- Raises insulin sensitivity
- Lowers blood sugar

Each of these benefits will be discussed below.

LDL Subclass B

The proper amount of exercise at the right intensity level increases LDL particle size and shifts distribution toward the A range. Although it is not well documented, combining this with a low-fat diet and weight loss may be enough to cause conversion to the intermediate or A subclass (especially for those with a 4 in their Apoprotein E test result). Particle size increases and distribution shifts *are* well documented and predictable, and when combined with effects of these other interventions, it is possible that a subclass B person can cross over into a lower risk zone. Even when this doesn't happen, reduction in small LDL particles such as LDL III levels will cause substantial reduction of risk. In addition, exercise induces chemical changes in the structure of the LDL subclass B particles that make them less susceptible to oxidation.

LDL Cholesterol Levels

The effect that exercise will have on LDL cholesterol levels is not as predictable as is the specific response of the LDL particle. Usually, LDL cholesterol remains fairly stable despite large amounts of exercise. The particle changes described above may be masked by an unchanged LDL cholesterol level.

Triglycerides

Of all the risk parameters, triglycerides probably respond most sensitively and immediately to exercise. There is a dose-dependent response. In the National Runners' Health Study, which looked at 10,000 male and 1,800 female runners, triglyceride levels fell on average almost half a mg/dl per mile run per week!

HDL Cholesterol and HDL2

This is where the most valuable benefits from metabolic exercise are. The effect of exercise on HDL and HDL2 levels is complex, and at least in part dependent upon concurrent diet and fat weight loss. Enough of the right kind of exercise will cause substantial changes in body makeup. Fat will be replaced by gains in muscle mass even without cutting calories. Consequently, HDL and HDL2 will rise without a measurable weight loss.

In men, the genetic predisposition for certain baseline levels of HDL and HDL2 will modulate the magnitude of the response to exercise. Men whose HDL levels were initially below average will experience smaller rises in levels versus men whose levels were initially above normal. Also, the changes in HDL cholesterol levels and HDL2 levels also may not be parallel. Many people will experience small or even no rises in their HDL cholesterol levels, while the HDL2 subfraction rises appreciably.

How high can your HDL cholesterol go?

Perhaps the best study looking at this question is the National Runners' Health Study. For every kilometer run per week, the average elevation was .14 mg/dl for the men and .13 for the women. Running twenty miles per week could boost your HDL by an average of 4 mg or about 10 percent of an average level. And with enough exercise, the right diet, and fat weight loss, you can push HDL2s to approach 100 percent—an enormous amplification of the effect of any rise of HDL cholesterol on reverse cholesterol transport.

In younger women runners on birth control pills, the dose-dependent HDL rise was lost. HDLs still rose, but not in the predictable manner, nor in the magnitude of the women not on pills. That's because of the alteration in the normal hormonal balance involving estrogen.

Diabetes, Insulin Sensitivity, and Blood Sugar

Metabolic conditioning sensitizes the muscles to insulin, amplifying its ability to transport glucose into the cell. This effect persists many hours after the exercise session. In addition, exercising muscles don't even need insulin in order to get that circulating sugar into them. The fat weight loss of exercise also improves insulin sensitivity. The net result can be very significant falls in circulating insulin levels, a rise in systemic insulin sensitivity, and a reduced or even eliminated reliance on medication to control a diabetic condition.

The Program: Choose Your Exercise Based on Your Risk

To design a good exercise program, you have to make an assessment of just what benefits you want from it. Your most prominent risk determines the intensity, frequency, and duration of your exercise. It is a question of emphasis, not exclusive categories. Serious mechanical cardiac benefits will be gained from a lower level exercise program, just as significant metabolic benefits will result from higher-level exercise.

You also have to assess how fit you are, because your fitness will determine at what level you can begin an exercise program,

Your Fitness Classification

		Age			
		20–29*	*30–39*	*40–49*	*50+*
Men	Superior	34–36	35–38	37–39	37–40
	Very good	37–40	39–41	40–42	41–43
	Good	41–42	42–43	43–44	44–45
	Fair	43–47	44–47	45–49	46–49
	Low	48–51	48–51	50–53	50–53
	Poor	52–59	52–59	54–60	54–62
Women	Superior	39–42	39–42	41–43	41–44
	Very good	43–44	43–45	44–45	45–47
	Good	45–46	46–47	46–47	48–49
	Fair	47–52	48–53	48–54	50–55
	Low	53–56	54–56	55–57	56–58
	Poor	57–66	57–66	58–67	59–66

*Numbers refer to 30-second heart rate.

Risk Factors Indicating a Need for Metabolic Conditioning

- LDL subclass B
- Low HDL cholesterol (including subclass As)
- Average HDL cholesterol with low HDL2
- Triglycerides in or above high normal range either as baseline or in response to a low-fat diet
- Obesity or BMI inappropriately high
- Undesirable waist-hip ratio
- Diabetes
- High LDL cholesterol (variable response)
- Chronic disability, illness, or being extremely unfit

Risk Factors Indicating a Need for Mechanical Conditioning

- Coronary artery disease *without* above risk factors
- Family history of premature coronary artery disease without identified risk factors
- High LDL cholesterol
- Subclass A with high Apoprotein B
- High blood pressure
- Smoking
- Elevated Lp(a)
- Elevated homocysteine
- Elevated fibrinogen

and whether you will have to build up to a target level. For example, someone with low HDL would want to exercise in the middle of Level 2. (See the table on page 190.) But if this person has never exercised before, then he needs to begin his program very low in Level 1 or perhaps even below Level 1, depending on his response to a fitness evaluation.

Your Fitness Classification

For people used to regular exercise, the guidelines depicted here are a model for fine-tuning your activities. If you do little or no exercise, you need to consider your approximate level of fitness compared to your peers. The most accurate way to do this is with a stress test. In this test, you exercise on a treadmill, gradually working up to your level of tolerance while attached to an electrocardiogram machine, which will detect any hidden cardiac abnormalities. Below is a list of people who should not start exercising until they have had this test:

Who Should Have a Stress Test

- Males over 40 years old who do not exercise
- Females over 50 years old who do not exercise
- Anyone who while doing any kind of physical activity develops chest pain or unusual shortness of breath
- Anyone with a family history of premature coronary artery disease
- Diabetics
- Smokers
- Asthmatics, or people with chronic lung disease
- Anyone with abnormal resting electrocardiograms, heart murmurs, or congenital heart problems
- Anyone with any kind of known heart disease

These tests frequently give false results, and they are not very informative in asymptomatic middle-aged people who are physically active. Still, if you fit one of these criteria, please see your doctor first. You should also consult your doctor if you have any fears about the safety of exercise. Often a good reason for a stress test is simply to gain peace of mind.

Even if the above list doesn't apply to you, you can find your fitness level with a simple test at home, using only a staircase or an 8-inch-high stool and a watch with a second hand. Make sure whatever you're using for the 8-inch-high step is stable. The exact height of 8 inches is important, too.

Start with your heart at normal resting pace—don't drink coffee, watch a horror movie, or do anything else to elevate your pulse. Every five seconds you should complete two steps up and down. This strict pacing is essential and might require some practice. The test requires you to perform this pace for three minutes. Then, exactly 30 seconds after you've finished, count your pulse for exactly another 30 seconds.

The chart on page 182 tells you where you fall relative to the general population. This is a very rough test with nowhere near the accuracy of a stress test or other formal fitness tests done in many health clubs; but it does give you an approximate idea of where it's safe to begin. Low and poor results mean that you need to enter any kind of exercise program very gradually and at a low intensity level. Fair to good means you're probably somewhere around average. Above that means you're fit and can enter an exercise program at a more ambitious intensity level. But in any case, these are very rough entry point guides. Ultimately how you feel while exercising will determine your progress.

At 50 percent of maximum heart rate, you should have absolutely no discomfort. At 60 to 70 percent of maximum heart rate, which corresponds to Level 1 in the chart on page 190, you should just start to feel as if you're working hard but far from uncomfortable. Level 2, however, should feel moderately stressful, with Level 3 being perceived as definitely hard to very hard work. Level 3 activity should be uncomfortable enough to suppress any desire, but not the ability, to talk.

The Exercise Continuum

Along the continuum of exercise from rest to highest tolerable intensity, there are changes in both mechanical and metabolic conditioning. Mechanically, the muscle becomes stronger as you move up the continuum. Metabolically, the ratio of sugar and fat (triglycerides) burned to produce energy changes as you move up the continuum. But while mechanical benefits increase as exercise intensity increases, the metabolic benefits you might need begin to fall off at a certain level of intensity. Where you

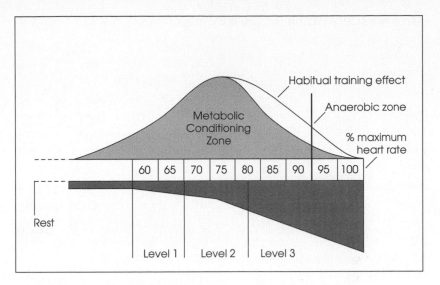

Figure 6. The Exercise Continuum

want to operate on the continuum will depend on your risks and what you want to accomplish.

The exercise continuum in the diagram in Figure 6 is based on maximum heart rate. Heart rate closely corresponds to oxygen consumption and the amount of energy you are expending while exercising. You can establish your maximum heart rate with a stress test, but you can make a fairly accurate estimate of it by subtracting your age from 220. Maximum heart rate (MHR) roughly corresponds to your maximum exercise capacity—that is, the maximum amount of energy you can consume in a given amount of time.

Mechanical Benefits on the Exercise Continuum

Mechanical benefits begin at about 60 percent of your maximum heart rate—indicated by Level 1 in Figure 6. As you go to 70 percent of MHR—Level 2 exercise—you are straining your muscles and beginning to experience more mechanical conditioning and its benefits. By Level 3, you are getting the full benefits of mechanical conditioning, and the more intense the exercise the better.

Metabolic Benefits on the Exercise Continuum

As you can see in Figure 6, metabolic conditioning doesn't increase in a straight line with the intensity of exercise. It increases through Level 2 exercise, but then begins to fall off.

Here's what's happening: You're always burning both fat (triglycerides) and sugar as you exercise, no matter what the level. At lower heart rate levels, the muscle is primarily using fat already circulating in the bloodstream as fuel. As the heart rate increases, and the intensity level increases, fuel must be burned faster, so fats are drawn from the internal supply of the muscle— they're closer than the fat in the blood. As we move beyond the 80 percent maximum heart rate level, much more sugar and less fat is being used. The sugar that is being used is drawn both from the circulation and from the internal muscle supply of sugar, called glycogen.

The key to reducing metabolic risk factors is to exercise at the level of intensity that will deplete the muscle cells' *internal* supply of fat. Why?

The answer lies in the enzyme called lipoprotein lipase, or LPL. LPL lines the walls of the blood vessels that supply the muscles, which is an enormous surface area. The muscles need LPL to strip off triglycerides from the lipid particles streaming in from the liver and intestines. These triglycerides replenish the muscles' internal triglyceride stores used up during exercise. The more these internal fats are depleted, the more intense the use of LPL becomes. The effect lasts about twenty-four hours after the exercise session ends. So if you exercise at the proper intensity for a long enough time every 24 hours or so, there will be a maximum depletion of triglycerides from the muscles, LPL stimulation will be more or less continuous, and you will produce a new metabolic state in your body.

This metabolic state you have produced dramatically reduces your risk factors. LDL particle size will move toward the less harmful larger size as triclycerides are removed from the circulation. HDLs and HDL2s will be generated. This powerful stimulation for HDL production accelerates the reabsorption of cholesterol plaques. The trick is to hit the right intensity level in your exercise to make all this happen, and to maintain that intensity long enough. If the exercise is too intense, then you use up too much glycogen, understimulating your LPL. If not intense

enough, then the muscles won't consume the internal fats, pre-
ferring to use circulating fats, and will fail to stimulate LPL after
exercise stops.

The shaded area at the top half of the exercise continuum
diagram in Figure 6 represents the level of LPL stimulation at any
given heart rate. This LPL stimulation is the metabolic conditioning effect we're focusing on. What's the magic intensity level?
Between 70 percent and 75 percent of your maximum heart rate,
which corresponds to Level 2 exercise. LPL stimulation peaks at
this point. As you can see, if you're exercising at Level 1 or Level
3, LPL is still stimulated, but you have to exercise longer for the
same metabolic effect.

There are metabolic effects in addition to LPL stimulation
that can be important in reducing risk factors. As you increase
your heart rate, the amount of glucose burned as fuel increases,
and this serves to deplete the muscles' glycogen store. Exercising
at higher heart rates, especially in Level 3, means the muscles are
primarily using sugar as an energy source, with fats serving as a
secondary fuel. Sugar is the high-octane fuel much more easily
converted into energy. So as an immediate energy source, the
muscles choose sugar over fat. This will deplete the glycogen in
the muscles, and replenishing it after exercise can become the
major focus of the body's metabolism.

This improves insulin metabolism. Normally insulin is required for a muscle cell to transport sugar from the blood into its
interior to recharge the glycogen stores. But with exercise, the
muscles become hyperresponsive to insulin, and during exercise
they don't even require insulin to draw the sugar in from the
bloodstream. Thus the amount of insulin you need declines, and
the body's carbohydrate-processing system becomes much more
efficient.

This has many benefits. An effect of lower insulin levels is to
release triglycerides from the body fat so that the muscle cells can
consume them. The liver is stimulated to generate blood sugar
rather than triclycerides, which get stored as fat. This all has a
favorable impact on the production of HDL and LDL particles.
But the level of glycogen depletion that is required to maximize
this effect usually means doing prolonged exercise at Level 3.
Most of us can't do that. This is why, in the exercise continuum
diagram, the metabolic benefits (as defined by the LPL effect,
not the insulin effect) decline as you move into Level 3—most of

us can't prolong Level 3 exercise long enough to achieve the maximum benefits of the changes in insulin metabolism.

Accomplished long-distance runners, cross-country skiers, marathoners, and other such athletes seem to enjoy the best of both worlds, with both high maximal exercise capacities and high HDLs, high HDL2, low triglycerides, and low LDL levels. The reason is that such athletes operate at high levels of intensity—Level 3—for extended periods of time. By doing so, they can maximally deplete the muscles' internal stores of both glycogen and triglycerides, thus stimulating LPL and improving insulin metabolism. They are not representative of the average exerciser, but they demonstrate the great potential benefit in both improved insulin metabolism and LPL stimulation one can receive if enough time is spent in Level 3. For most of us, the primary metabolic benefits will come from LPL stimulation, which occurs much more efficiently at more reasonable levels of exercise.

Calories and Exercise

But how can you determine your level of exercise? Since exercise level is determined by intensity, you need a practical measure of intensity. Measuring the number of calories used in a given period of time is one method, and it has the advantage of being usable, regardless of the activity. A calorie is a unit of energy. You can ingest a calorie, and you can burn a calorie. All exercise can be easily translated into calories, and we can talk about calories per minute, per hour, per week; or we can talk about calories per linear distance. This allows someone who participates in multiple sports to understand how different types of exercise, such as swimming, are equivalent to other types, such as running or playing tennis.

If you weigh 150 pounds, you use about 100 calories for every mile you run. You use about 400 calories for every mile of swimming and about 40 calories per mile cycling. You can then know that 12½ miles of cycling, 5 miles of running, or 1¼ miles of swimming give you the same workout. A table at the end of this chapter lists a number of common sports with their calorie equivalents for a person of about 160 pounds. The more you weigh, the higher these calorie counts rise.

Studies have shown that in middle-aged people, protection against heart disease requires a minimum intensity level of about 400 calories an hour, somewhat less for those who are older, and more for those younger. The rate of 400 calories per hour is the lower limit of the metabolic conditioning zone, or Level 1 exercise on the exercise continuum.

Your age determines your threshold for getting into this zone of exercise. This has been demonstrated by studies showing substantial HDL increases for older people engaged in slower paced exercise. The numbers in the table below are average values. If you are doing 2,000 calories or more of exercise per week at the minimum intensity for your age and not seeing improvements in risk factors, move up to a higher intensity.

Exercise Intensity Levels

Age	Intensity Threshold for Metabolic Conditioning (calories)	Equivalent Run/Walk Pace (mph)
20	490	4.9
25	450	4.5
30	440	4.4
35	410	4.1
40	400	4
45	380	3.8
50	350	3.5
55	330	3.3
60	300	3
65	280	2.8
70	250	2.5

Heart Rate and Exercise Intensity

Caloric expenditure, useful as it is, is still only an estimate. Measuring heart rate provides even more accurate information about just how hard your body is working.

Use the table on pages 193–194 as a guide to your fitness level. You can find your target heart rate using the following table. People with low fitness should start in Level 1 or below, people with "fair" to "good" fitness in lower Level 2, and "very good" to "superior" in upper Level 2. People with "poor" fitness scores should actually start below Level 1 and work up.

Target Heart Rates and Exercise Levels for Different Ages

Age	Max Heart Rate (MHR)	60% MHR	65% MHR	70% MHR	77% MHR	80% MHR	85% MHR	90% MHR
20	200	120	130	140	150	160	170	180
22	198	119	129	139	149	158	168	178
24	196	118	127	137	147	157	167	176
26	194	116	126	136	146	155	165	175
28	192	115	125	134	144	154	163	173
30	190	114	123	133	143	152	162	171
32	188	113	122	132	141	150	160	170
34	186	112	121	130	140	149	158	167
36	184	110	120	129	138	147	156	166
38	182	109	118	127	137	146	155	164
40	180	108	117	126	135	144	153	162
42	178	107	116	125	134	142	151	160
46	176	196	114	123	132	141	150	159
48	174	104	113	122	131	139	148	157
50	172	103	112	120	129	138	146	155
52	170	102	111	119	128	136	145	153
54	168	101	109	118	126	134	142	151
56	166	100	108	116	125	133	141	150
58	164	98	107	115	123	131	140	148
60	162	97	105	113	122	130	138	146
62	160	96	104	112	120	128	136	144
64	158	95	103	110	119	126	134	142
66	156	94	101	109	117	125	133	140
		Level 1		Level 2			Level 3	

For example, if you are a forty-year-old with fair fitness, then you should start low in Level 1 and have a target heart rate in your first weeks of exercise of 108. If metabolic conditioning is the goal, then over the subsequent months, you should build to a heart rate that falls in the Level 2 zone, somewhere between 126 and 135. Or if you are a forty-year-old woman with an average fitness score who has targeted Level 3 as a desired range then you would start at Level 2, somewhere between 126 and 135, and gradually build up over the subsequent weeks so that you are exercising at a heart rate higher than 144. A safe rate of progress is to increase the heart rate at which you exercise by 5 percent to 10 percent per week. People with coronary artery disease should progress even more slowly.

By targeting the risk factors that most concern you, you can decide whether you need to emphasize mechanical or metabolic improvement from your exercise. There are people who may feel they are somewhere in the middle. The benefits of metabolic and mechanical conditioning can *both* be maximized if you have the time and the physical resilience to exercise for two to three hours a day at Level 3, or above 80 percent of your maximum heart rate. But for most people, compromises must be made. If you look at Figure 6, the exercise continuum diagram, you see the answer to this dilemma. At around the 75 percent maximum heart rate point, there's an overlap of the two conditioning zones. If you feel your needs for reducing risk factors require equal portions of both kinds of exercise, this is the optimum level of intensity around which you should build your workouts.

I particularly recommend this target for people who already have active coronary artery disease and who have significant metabolic risks that are not adequately or comfortably controlled with medications. Under the direction of a gradual cardiac rehabilitation program most people can attain this goal, and almost all people in their forties and fifties with premature coronary artery disease can.

If you're primarily interested in lowering circulating metabolic risk factors, you must maximize your muscles' reliance on internal fat supplies for fuel by exercising in Level 2. As you push exercise intensity higher into Level 2, you also train your muscles not to use as much glucose for any given level of intensity. This is the "metabolic training effect." Fats are used more efficiently at higher levels of exercise intensity while reliance on glycogen—sugars—falls. Consequently, high levels of LPL stimulation are achieved at exercise levels that would be too intense for an untrained person. Thus a training program widens the peak metabolic conditioning effect on LPL into the lower Level 3 region. This allows maximal LPL stimulation while increasing the mechanical benefits of exercise—the best of both worlds.

Duration

The mechanical effects of exercise precede the desired metabolic effects on fat metabolism by 20 to 30 minutes. That's because muscles use almost exclusively glucose before they are warmed up. In other words, if you exercise only 20 or 30 minutes, you help your cardiovascular system, but you don't stimulate LPL. So if your cardiac risk is primarily defined in terms of metabolic risk factors, you don't get much out of 20 or 30 minutes of exercise.

In carefully controlled studies of exercisers, those exercising at the lower intensity levels—around 60 percent to 70 percent of maximum heart rate for longer periods—enjoyed high elevations of HDL, HDL2, LDL particle size increase, and weight loss. In fact, depending on the study design, many of the people with the greatest decline in risk factors showed minimal improvements in their mechanical conditioning. These people did improve their *endurance,* their capacity for sustained lower levels of performance at Level 1 or Level 2, because they trained their muscles to rely mostly on fats. But for short-term, more intense aerobic exercise, their conditioning was not nearly as good.

Short duration (less than 40 minutes) exercise at Level 3 anatomically and physiologically strengthens the heart against the *effects* of atherosclerosis. Prolonged—45 minutes or more— sessions of metabolic exercise at Level 2 or Level 1 reduce the metabolic factors *causing* atherosclerosis. For most people, an exercise program must be fine-tuned to provide more metabolic or cardiovascular benefit, depending on needs. Your exercise program has to be balanced, and compromises have to be made.

The definitive study on exercise duration is one done in 1992 in Heidelberg, Germany. People with coronary artery disease who were placed on an exercise program had their atherosclerotic lesions measured before and after the program. They were compared to a control group not on an exercise regimen.

About half of all the patients, control and treated alike, demonstrated no changes in the extent of their disease. Practically all of the other control patients got worse. The other patients on the aggressive exercise regimen, however, actually demonstrated arrest or melting of their atherosclerotic lesions. No patient who exercised less than 1,600 calories a week demonstrated melting of the cholesterol plaque, and practically all of those who did reduce lesions required exercise volumes greater than 2,200 calories per week—that's 22 miles of running. And the minimally effective intensity level was 400 calories an hour. In their follow-up, the researchers found that these hard-won benefits could be maintained with an exercise volume of about 1,800 calories a week.

The minimum volume of exercise to increase mechanical cardiovascular fitness was about 1,400 calories per week. No one in the study demonstrated an appreciable increase in mechanical cardiovascular fitness below this level.

So how much you exercise is just as important as the intensity level. This is where defining exercise in terms of calories is so helpful. The daily calorie expenditure isn't as important as the total calories of continuous exercise accumulated over a week. Level 1 and Level 2 exercisers need a minimum of 2,000 calories. Level 3 exercisers who are not as concerned with metabolic effects should do a minimum of 1,500 calories. However, for Level 3 exercise, it takes at least 20 minutes before the muscles get warmed up enough to draw on fats for fuel. For many Level 3 exercisers this is of no consequence, but if you're at this level and want the same kind of metabolic benefits that lower exercise levels will deliver, you shouldn't count the first 20 minutes of each exercise session in your weekly calorie count. This may mean extending a 30-minute workout to 45 minutes or an hour.

An alternative is to slow down from Level 3 but exercise even longer. In the upper range of Level 2 or the lower range of Level 3, glucose is still being recruited to provide a significant portion of the muscles' fuel. Thus to deplete the muscles' fat, you need to extend the duration of the workout to more than an hour instead of the usual thirty- or forty-minute session. You'll get the mechanical benefits of high intensity while still supercharging LPL, but it takes more time.

Below are three different exercise plans for three forty-year-olds with different levels of fitness and different risk profiles. In each case, the exercise program is designed to counter the individual risk factors.

Level 1, Exercise Week for 40-Year-Old Novice Exerciser

LDL subclass B, low HDL, overweight, BMI = 29
2,100 calories per week of exercise

Monday	Tuesday	Wednesday	Thursday	Friday	Saturday	Sunday
Walk 3 miles in 45–60 minutes. Heart rate: 108–117	Same	Same	Same	Rest	Walk 6 miles in 1½ to 2 hours.	Walk 3 miles in 45–60 minutes.

Level 2, Exercise Week for 40-Year-Old Experienced Exerciser

LDL subclass B, low HDL, High triglycerides, BMI = 27
2,600 calories

Monday	Tuesday	Wednesday	Thursday	Friday	Saturday	Sunday
Jog 4 miles in 45 minutes. Heart rate: 125–135	Same	Swim 1 mile in 45 minutes. Heart rate: 125–134	Run 2 miles in 15 minutes. Heart rate: 145–150	Swim 1 mile in 45 minutes. Heart rate: 125–135	Jog 6 miles in 1½ hours. Heart rate: 125–135	Singles tennis, 1½ hours.

Level 3, Exercise Week for 40-Year-Old Experienced Exerciser

LDL subclass A, average HDL, high HDL2, BMI = 24
2,400 calories

Monday	Tuesday	Wednesday	Thursday	Friday	Saturday	Sunday
Rest	Run 4 miles in 30 minutes. Heart rate: 145–165	Rest	Cycle 20 miles in 1 hour. Heart rate: 145–165	Rest	Run 4 miles in 30 minutes. Heart rate: 145–165	Cycle 20 miles in 1 hour. Heart rate: 145–165

Frequency

After an exercise session, LPL levels remain revved up for about 24 hours, so for optimal metabolic effects, exercising every day, or almost every day, is best. Most of the other hormonal changes that are working to your advantage are also temporary, dwindling away after 24–48 hours.

For mechanical cardiovascular conditioning only, on the other hand, it's actually beneficial to have a day of rest between workouts, especially if you are high in Level 3. Your 1,500- to 2,000-calorie week of workouts should be divided into four sessions of about 30 minutes to 40 minutes each.

In order to realize the benefits, your exercise session must be *continuous*. Spreading 5- or 10-minute sessions throughout the day (climbing a few flights of stairs every few hours) might result in some cardiovascular conditioning benefits, but it will do almost nothing for metabolic adaptations.

Exercise and Eating

Performing well in a sport at any level of exercise requires an adequate supply of carbohydrates. This is true even when you're exercising at a level where primarily fats are being used as fuel. That's because when a muscle contracts, it uses a mix of fuels— fat and sugar. The slower the contraction, the greater the proportion of fat used to energize it. But sugar is still necessary. Even when you exercise at level 1, some of the muscle's glycogen reserve gets used up, and at level 2, even more sugar is burned. This adds up, day after day, even at lower levels of exercise. So you must eat carbohydrates after exercise in order to fully replenish the lost glycogen.

Glycogen depletion makes the muscles slow down, reducing their energy output. At low levels of exercise intensity, the least efficient but most plentiful of all possible fuels, which are the fats circulating in your bloodstream, are used to fuel the muscles. The lack of carbohydrate in the fuel mix forces the muscle to perform at a level so low that it bypasses its own fat stores. This means LPL isn't intensely stimulated because it doesn't have to rebuild those fat stores after the exercise session. And stimulation of LPL is the mechanism for risk reduction.

Those currently advocating eating fats for sports and weight loss are trying to outsmart this system. It doesn't work. Even at Level 1 exercise levels, if a person is going to exercise every day for an hour or so, a low-carbohydrate diet will induce fatigue, missed days, and lower intensity levels over time.

So how do you eat? The 30-55-15 breakdown of the amount of fat, carbohydrate, and protein of the recommended low-fat diet is fine. Marathoners and the like will probably do better with 20-65-15 or even 15-65-20.

In addition, it's very important to replenish a glycogen reserve during the optimal glycogen replenishment period, which is in the first four hours after exercise. It is here, finally, where all those high-sugar, low-fat foods blacklisted in the diet chapter play a healthy role. Rapidly available simple carbohydrates (also found in fruit) replace expended muscle glycogen most efficiently.

By knowing how many calories you've burned, you can approximate how much carbohydrate you should eat in the 4 to 6 hours after a session, or should add to your total diet. At Level 1, your fuel mix is about 75:25, fat:sugar, so if you used 500 calories, replenishing just 125 of them with added dietary sugars should be adequate. Let the rest of the total energy deficit come from your body fat.

At Level 2, the fuel mix in the trained muscle is about 60:40, fat:sugar and at Level 3, more like 20:80, fat:sugar. It's the Level 3 people who are obviously most concerned with carbohydrate loading, especially when engaged in endurance levels of exercise.

These numbers are approximate, and you have to experiment. You'll know if you're on target because you will lose a small amount of weight, not feel hungry, and not notice unusual fatigue or decreased ability to exercise. If you do experience any of these last two, you may not be eating enough carbohydrates.

You shouldn't have a high carbohydrate meal that will get absorbed within two hours before exercise starts. Doing so will keep insulin levels high early in the workout, and insulin prevents fat usage. And since the earlier meal's carbohydrates have probably been cleared from the blood already, the muscle is forced to use its own carbohydrates for even longer than the warm-up period.

Exercise should be started on an empty stomach to minimize insulin levels and maximize fat use. Alternatively, you can eat a carbohydrate load *immediately* before starting exercise. Once muscles are active, they actually don't need insulin to absorb glucose. However, this makes many people feel uncomfortable, even sick. For those who tolerate it, it's a very convenient way to minimize the initial depletion of glycogen that occurs at the beginning of every exercise session while minimizing the interferences with fat usage. This pays off later at the end of very long endurance sessions because more glycogen has been spared to sustain you toward the end of the session.

Exercise and Blood Clotting

Exercise has as profound a beneficial effect on the blood clotting system as it does on circulating lipid factors. It is an extremely potent way to increase the body's ability to dissolve blood clots in the arteries. But just as with lipid factors, the kind of exercise you do is crucial to obtaining the benefit.

In a study done in Bethesda, Maryland, sedentary men were compared to serious recreational joggers and marathon runners. There was a graded increase in each group, determined by their physical conditioning, in their ability to dissolve clots. The higher the person's performance level, the more potent the clot-dissolving capacity. Though the joggers were very fit, the marathoners were fitter and enjoyed substantially more benefit.

Fibrinolysis, the term for this clot-dissolving phenomenon, is a system that seems to have a thirst for exercise. It can't get too much of it. Wherever it has been studied, the people with the most supercharged fibrinolytic systems were the ones with the highest work capacities. Men exercising at a moderate aerobic pace increase their ability to dissolve blood clots by a factor of five, but when they accelerate beyond Level 3, they raise their ability to dissolve blood clots by a factor of 45. Women have less dramatic responses, but they still benefit from higher intensity. When you engage in intense exercise you actually start to dissolve the blood clots forming on your plaques. We know that for a fact, because in these same studies, tests for dissolved clot fragments are positive. Obviously, the more time you spend in Level 2 and Level 3 exercise, the more atherosclerotic meltdown you get.

The exercise effects on the conditioning of blood aren't limited to fibrinolysis. Exercise causes the volume of plasma in the circulation to increase. This protects against the effects of plaque limiting the blood flow. It dilutes the red blood cells; and while this may sound like a bad thing, it really is advantageous. Diluted blood flows more freely and faster, resulting in a net *increase* in oxygen delivery to the cells. Though there may be fewer red cells in any given volume of blood, the faster flow brings more red cells to the tissues for any given period of time, and with them, more oxygen.

These are effects with staying power. They are adaptations the body makes to the repetitive stress of the intense appetite for oxygen caused by vigorous exercise. As with fibrinolysis, it is at Level 3 where these changes are most dramatic.

Because the effect of intense exercise on blood clotting is so impressive, moving up from Level 1 to Level 2 is all the more important. Those engaged in Level 2 and Level 3 exercise should undertake interval training, which means jumping into the next exercise level for as long as tolerated, recovering, and then doing it again. Most experts on heart disease and exercise recommend against this, because of the fear that it will itself cause a heart attack. This is perfectly reasonable fear, and that's why intervals of maximal exercise are not for everyone. But if you are young or an experienced high-level exerciser, it is appropriate to incorporate one or two limited sessions a week of structured interval training, or, even better, a brief period of maximal exertion in most of your workouts. People with the highest exercise capacities produce the most intense stimulus for fibrinolysis. The importance of developing a supercharged fibrinolytic system cannot be overemphasized.

Exercise and Wellness

Finally, exercise has many benefits that are not directly connected to cardiac health. Exercise—at the right threshold of intensity—causes a release of endorphins, generating a general sense of well being and counteracting stress. This requires at least Level 2 exercise for 45 minutes to an hour.

In physical training studies of middle-aged men, regular exercise could completely block in them the physiologically normal deterioration of maximal exercise capacity over the next 10 years. This kind of time travel is possible even when you think you may be too far gone to be salvaged. It's been found that even 60- and 70-year-olds can achieve the physical performance levels of their 40- and 50-year-old counterparts if they are engaged in a systematic, gradual exercise program.

Noncardiac Benefits of Exercise

- Increased muscle mass and strength
- Blocking of age-related decline in muscle mass
- Decreased body fat
- Joint flexibility
- Preserved lung capacity
- Facilitated neuron transmissions
- Increased brain activity
- Resistance to depression
- Resistance to common forms of cancer, especially colon and breast
- Conservation of bone mass
- Increased immune function

Caloric Equivalents of Time-Measured Activities*

Activity	Hours Representing 2,000 Calories	Intensity: Calories per Hour
Badminton	5	400
Basketball	3½	511
Boxing	2¼	888
Canoe leisure	11	181
Canoe racing	4¾	421
Circuit training:		
Universal	4¼	470
Nautilus	5½	363
free weights	5¾	347
Climbing Hills:		
no load	4	500
10 lbs.	3¾	533
20 lbs.	3½	571
40 lbs.	3¼	615
Dancing:		
aerobic (medium)	4¾	421
aerobic (intense)	3⅔	555
ballroom	9½	210
contemporary	4¾	421
Downhill Skiing (moderate)	4½	450
Downhill Skiing (expert level)	3⅓	600
Field Hockey	3⅔	555
Football	3¾	533
Horse riding:		
gallop	3½	571
trot	4½	444
walking	12	166
Judo	2½	800
Jumping rope:		
70 RPM	3	666
80 RPM	3	666
125 RPM	2¾	727
145 RPM	2½	800
Racquetball	2¾	727
Forestry:		
Ax chopping (fast)	1⅔	1,250
Ax chopping (slow)	5¾	347
Sawing	4	500
Gardening:		
digging	9	222

continues

*155-pound person

Caloric Equivalents of Time-Measured Activities*
Continued

Activity	Hours Representing 2,000 Calories	Intensity: Calories per Hour
hedging	6½	307
mowing	4¼	470
raking	9	222
Gymnastics	7½	266
Scuba diving:		
considerable motion	1¾	1,142
moderate motion	2⅓	869
Snowshoeing (soft snow)	3	666
Squash	2⅓	869
Table tennis	7¼	275
Tennis	4½	444
Volleyball	9¾	205

*155-pound person

Sports Measured by Distance*

	2,000 Calories	Calories/ Mile	400 Calories/ Hour
Canoeing	50 miles	40	10 mph
Roller or ice skating	45 miles	44	9 mph
Cycling	50 miles	40	10 mph
Cross-country skiing	11 miles	180	2.2 mph
Running	20 miles	100	4 mph (15-minute mile)
Swimming	5 miles	400	1 mph
Walking	26 miles	78	5 mph

*155-pound person

15

Step Ten:
Consider the Right
Medication for Your Type

It's nice to think that assiduous attention to diet, weight, and exercise will always be enough to eliminate risks, but sometimes it just isn't. For many of the risk factors of heart disease, medications are needed, and they are often needed in combination. The choice of the appropriate therapy is as individualized as every other aspect of coronary artery risk intervention. There are no generic prescriptions that can be used by everyone.

What Do the Drugs Do?

Goal	Active Drugs
Conversion of LDL subclass B to A	niacin
	fibrates
	resins
	estrogen
Reduction of LDL cholesterol level	statins
	resins
	niacin
	fibrates (unreliably)
Elevation of HDL and HLD2	niacin
	fibrates
	estrogen
Reduction of triglycerides	Fibrates
	niacin
	atrovastatin
Reduction of fibrinogen	fibrates
Homocysteine	folate
	B_6
Lp(a)	niacin
	estrogens

Niacin

Niacin is as close to a magic bullet as there is for treating the predominant risk factors of coronary artery disease. Natural vitamin B_3, nicotinic acid, is a reliable weapon for converting LDL subclass B to A, a conversion very difficult to make with lifestyle changes alone.

Niacin is also the most reliable drug for raising resistantly low HDL and HDL2 levels. An effective dose of Niacin can raise HDL by 20 percent to 40 percent and can increase HDL2 percentage by as much as 100 percent. The drug is also an effective reducer of triglyceride levels. And finally, short of hormone therapy, niacin is about the only treatment currently available for high Lp(a).

How does niacin work? Niacin participates in many of the fundamental energy cycles of the body. Taken in large enough doses, it inhibits the liver's ability to produce VLDLs, the triglyceride-laden parent of the LDL particle. At the same time, it stimulates the synthesis of HDL precursors destined to become HDL2 and HDL3.

Apart from its direct actions upon the liver, niacin suppresses the mobilization of triglycerides from adipose tissue and thereby interrupts this usually constant infusion of triglycerides into the liver, where they become incorporated into the VLDL particles.

Side Effects

Unfortunately, niacin has side effects that make it complicated to prescribe and difficult to take. Therapeutic doses of niacin can cause alarming flushing, feelings of heat, itching, headaches, palpitations, and panic. However, in the great majority of cases these problems can be eliminated by using the proper dosing method, increasing doses gradually, and taking it with meals and aspirin. There is also a new preparation, discussed below, that helps eliminate these side effects.

Other side effects are nausea, heartburn, cramps, and aggravation of chronic stomach problems, such as ulcers and gastritis. If you have these kinds of serious problems you need an alternative to niacin.

Perhaps the most ominous side effect of niacin is silent: hepatitis. Therapeutic doses of niacin commonly will cause mild elevation of liver enzymes. This is a sign of possible liver damage. Stopping the drug for a few weeks or reducing the dose can relieve this problem. In rare cases, serious resistant hepatitis is produced. Because of these liver effects, people on therapeutic doses of niacin require periodic laboratory tests to determine their liver function.

Other serious complications are aggravation of gout, aggravation of a tendency for the heart to beat rapidly and cause palpitations, and diabetes. Oddly, niacin is the most effective, single treatment of all of the lipid disorders that come with diabetes: high triglycerides, low HDL, LDL subclass B. Because of this, it isn't justified to withhold this vital drug from the diabetic; most will tolerate it and will benefit enormously as a result. But again, as with the liver tissue, use of niacin with diabetes requires careful evaluation and follow-up by your doctor.

In the hands of experienced doctors, niacin doses can be reduced appreciably and their side effects avoided when used in combination with fibrates, resins, or both. The three drugs act in synergy, and the reduced doses of each minimize side effects.

Niacin combined with statins can be beneficial for both subclass A and B people. For subclass As with low HDLs, the addition of niacin will increase HDL and further reduce LDL cholesterol. For the subclass B person who has converted to subclass A with niacin but still has a high LDL cholesterol, the addition of the statin is a perfect complement.

As we have seen, there are some very inconvenient and even frightening aspects to taking niacin. About one in three people will not tolerate the doses required to treat their LDL subclass or Lp(a) problem and will need alternate therapy, or an emphasis on eliminating all other more treatable risk factors. But for the majority, who can tolerate niacin, the benefits are great, since niacin can convert a high-risk person into virtually a *no* risk person.

Doses and Preparations

The RDA of vitamin B_3, niacin, is 20 mg. A typical high-potency vitamin might have 30 mg. Typically, it takes from 1,000 to 2,000 mgs to change LDL subclass, triglycerides, and HDL. To affect Lp(a) levels may require three times these doses.

Until very recently, using niacin required elaborate dosing protocols to minimize side effects. But a new form of niacin, Niaspan, is now available, and almost everyone can use it without the most annoying side effect, flushing. Niaspan is a form of extended-release niacin that works much better than older versions.

The effective dose of Niaspan, as with the older formulations, must be built up over the course of weeks or even months The drug comes in a convenient dose pack, and you take one pill each night just before sleep, and preferably after dinner. Most people report some very mild flushing in the first few weeks.

And it works. Finally, after years of struggling with this drug, we can offer anyone whose lethal risk factors require it the most effective treatment in our armamentarium. Niacin may prove to be one of the most dramatic lifesavers in the history of medicine.

Statins

There are five of these drugs now available: lovastatin (Mevacor), simvastatin (Zocor), fluvastatin (Lescor), pravastatin (Pravachol), and atrovastatin (Lipitor).

Currently statins are the glamour drugs of preventive cardiology. They enjoy the benefit of great press from three large studies that used them to treat high cholesterol. But they are often not used properly. They are being prescribed for LDL cholesterol reduction indiscriminately, as a result at least half of those receiving them don't benefit. Why? Because statins don't convert subclass B to subclass A.

In addition, for the people who can respond to them, they are not being prescribed in doses that lower LDL cholesterol to the goal levels described in chapter 8. A recent study of people being treated by primary care physicians revealed that 62 percent did not have proper drug dosing or effective LDL cholesterol reduction.

Statins act by inhibiting the liver enzyme that creates cholesterol. LDL particle production is reduced, and LDL receptors become hungrier and thus more effective at clearing cholesterol.

The key point here is that statins either reduce *all* LDL particles more or less uniformly or they preferentially reduce the large, buoyant A particles. That's why LDL cholesterol levels fall—there's less cholesterol around. That's also why Apoprotein B levels fall; there are fewer particles around. But a subclass B remains a subclass B.

By reducing total LDL particle numbers and total amounts of LDL cholesterol, the subclass B person who started out with elevated levels is better off but still at high risk. Such people do well on a combination of a statin and niacin or another of the "B-particle drugs."

While they are second line therapy for the subclass B patient with elevated LDL cholesterol levels that are resistant to niacin, statins are the first-line drug for reducing subclass A LDL cholesterol levels. For the subclass A person, these truly are miracle drugs if used aggressively. Many people see modest rises in HDL and falls in triglycerides, but it has not been shown that those effects are meaningful when induced by these drugs.

To illustrate this point, the newest of the statins, atrovastatin (Lipitor) has resulted in dramatic falls in triglyceride levels and rises in HDL levels. However, there was no observable change in the LDL particle distribution of those who are subclass B. To date, no statin has shown activity against this problem.

The appreciable rises in HDL levels sometimes seen with the statins seem to be a great benefit. It is known that simvastatin can raise HDL2 levels, but we don't have sufficient knowledge about all the effects this kind of drug can have on HDL particles.

It has recently been found that statins stabilize the fragile outer canopy of the lipid-rich plaque, thus protecting it from rupture. Pravachol does this best, and there is some evidence simvastatin does it, too.

Average Expected Changes (mg/dl)

	LDL Decrease	HDL Increase	TG Decrease	Daily Cost (in dollars)
Lovastatin	32	8	15	2–8
Simvastatin	33	10	15	2–4
Pravastatin	29	7	17	2–3
Fluvastatin	30	7	11	1–3
Atrovastatin	48	22	28	2–7

Side Effects

These drugs are tolerated very well. Their ease of use and few side effects are keys to their popularity. There is a small incidence of liver toxicity, which responds to discontinuation or reduction of the dose. Stomach upset, inflammation of the muscles, skin rashes, and sleep disturbances can all occur, but they are uncommon and easily prevented or treated by watching symptoms carefully.

Fibrates (Fibric Acid Derivatives)

Fibrates (called gemfibrozil or Lopid) exert their effects on lipid levels by stimulating LPL. In a sense, they're the pharmacological supplement of exercise. By stimulating LPL, VLDL particles are reduced and triglyceride levels fall. Generally, the higher the triglycerides, the more they fall. Fibrates are most effective when triglycerides are over 200. Also as a result of the LPL activity, HDL cholesterol levels and HDL2 percentages increase, though not reliably.

Fibrates are, therefore, drugs for treating high triglycerides, low HDL in the presence of triglyceride levels over 200, and for converting LDL subclass B to A, also in the presence of triglyceride levels above 200. In this latter context, fibrates can substitute for niacin.

But the effects this drug has on LDL cholesterol levels—as opposed to subclass—are much more problematic. When used to treat a high triglyceride level in the presence of normal LDL cholesterol levels, the latter may rise appreciably while the former falls. By contrast, people with elevated LDL cholesterol may see an improvement in this value. Generally, these effects are secondary, and fibrates are not first-line therapy for elevated LDL cholesterol.

Finally, fibrates are the only drugs that can reliably reduce fibrinogen concentrations and some of the other circulatory elements of the blood that promote clot formation.

Side Effects

Unless absolutely necessary I don't recommend that people with gallbladder disease and gallstones take these drugs. For others, Lopid is well tolerated. The most common complaints are gastrointestinal: nausea, cramps, and flatulence are fairly common but subside once the person becomes accustomed to the drug.

There is a very small incidence of muscle inflammation, a side effect similar to the statins. When fibrates are used in combination with statins, as they often are, you should be alert for unusual muscle aches and pains that persist for more than a day or two.

Resins

Colestipol (Colestid) and cholestyramine (Questran), the bile acid binding resins, are among the oldest anticholesterol medications. They act by binding bile secreted by the gallbladder. Bile is important because it's full of cholesterol discarded by the liver. The problem is that much of this cholesterol gets reabsorbed when it reaches the intestine. The resins break this cycle by forcing its elimination in the stool. By eliminating this inflow of cholesterol to the liver, the liver's overloaded cholesterol receptors get hungry again and can more effectively clear the circulation of more cholesterol.

Another reaction by the liver to this decreased inflow of cholesterol is to increase production of cholesterol. That's how the liver tries to circumvent the therapeutic effects of the resin. Therefore resins are often used not as single agents but in combination with statins. Since they act in perfect synergy, the doses of each can be reduced often by as much as half, and therefore, so can the side effects.

Resins reduce LDL cholesterol and can reduce LDL particle numbers. The LDL particle reduction in the subclass A person will be mainly reducing the large A particles. When resins are given to the subclass B person, the small dense particles are primarily reduced. It's also been found that resins are much more able to reduce the number of subclass B particles than subclass A particles, so these drugs result in greater reductions of LDL cholesterol in the subclass B person than in subclass A. For a subclass B person who just can't tolerate niacin, resins are an alternative, either alone or combined with a statin or fibrates.

Otherwise, a resin-and-niacin combination is an excellent choice for the subclass B problem, and when used in combination, the dosages of each can be reduced.

Side Effects

Side effects are mainly the result of intestinal irritation: cramps, bloating, belching, and especially, constipation. These can usually be averted with reduced doses in combination regimens. Sometimes, however, this doesn't work, and the drug must be discontinued.

Since resins are chemical binders, they can make other medications or vitamins you may be taking ineffective. So don't take them at the same time.

Antioxidants: Vitamins C and E

The Cambridge Heart Attack and Antioxidant Study (rather ominously called CHAOS) has established the importance of vitamin E in the regimen of *every* person at risk for heart disease. Eight hundred units per day resulted in a 56 percent reduction in nonfatal heart attacks over only a year and a half in 2,000 patients. This is powerful testament to the power of LDL oxidation to create havoc.

Vitamin E binds to the LDL particle and alters its chemical structure to make it much more resistant to oxidation. But vitamin E itself gets used up in the process and needs an antioxidant itself. That's where vitamin C comes in, preserving the antioxidant efficiency of vitamin E.

So the two go together. Vitamin E should be taken as 800 units either all at once or in divided doses. Vitamin C, on the other hand, should be time released or taken in divided doses two or three times a day with a total dose of 1,000 to 1,500 mgs daily. The reason vitamin C doses should be split is that it is rapidly eliminated by the kidneys. Unlike vitamin E, which binds to the fats in cells and particle membranes, vitamin C doesn't hang around in the circulation, so a constant renewal of its level optimizes its effects.

Foods high in vitamin E are olive oil, sunflower oil, fortified cereals (look at the label), and wheat germ. Don't rely on foods, however, for vitamin E. You should take supplements. Each day I begin my day with my "longevity cocktail": one aspirin, 800 units of vitamin E, and the first dose of 500 units of vitamin C. I strongly recommend this to everyone (except those who shouldn't be taking aspirin). The added theoretical benefit of taking these two vitamins is that they will also contribute to the muscle building and recovery process of repetitive exercise.

While antioxidants can be considered a helpful option for many people, there are groups whose risk factors make them prone to LDL oxidation, and they should definitely be on a routine of vitamin E and C supplements: LDL subclass B, high Lp(a), low HDL, LDL subclass A with heart disease.

Medicines are not a panacea. They are to be resorted to if reaching proper weight and adopting the right exercise and diet habits have not attained your risk reduction goals. The exceptions are those people who already have coronary artery disease or extremely high LDL levels and other risk factors. Even in such cases, for medicines to work effectively, they must be introduced as an adjunct to, and not a substitute for, these basic lifestyle measures.

Afterword

I have drawn a picture of heart disease based on our most up-to-date understanding of the disorder, a picture that may be quite different from your current understanding. Heart disease is a much more serious danger—and yet at the same time a much more preventable disease—than you may have imagined.

Atherosclerosis begins when you are a child, and by puberty children should be taking measures against it. This is a lesson you have learned, and now you should teach your children.

You've also learned that the traditional concepts for determining who is at risk for coronary artery disease actually miss most of the people who will go on to have heart attacks. The simple advice to "avoid red meat and cheese" and "keep your cholesterol low" is not enough to ensure protection. We know much more now about how to prevent heart disease, and you can tailor a program that matches your own individual risks and metabolism.

You now know how to identify risk. The first step is to gather the essential information. Some people will want the entire panoply of available tests; others will be satisfied with fewer. But everyone should at the very least establish his or her LDL level and subclass in any lipid profile and carefully examine the history of heart disease in his or her family.

You also now know how to take action against heart disease. If you start early enough, many risk factors can be disarmed without medication. In its early stages, atherosclerosis is as vulnerable as it is insidious. Diet and exercise can melt it away and prevent it from returning. But even diet and exercise programs have to be tailored to the individual. Generic advice applied to everyone will not do much good and can do considerable harm. Almost every identified risk has a lifestyle antidote—but you have to know what each risk is, and what antidote should be applied.

Eating right and exercising regularly are essential to healthy longevity. There is no easy way around this. But you have to know how to eat right and how to exercise in order to reap the benefits. Again, what is right for one person will not be right for another.

Certain medications have now been proven to be lifesaving clinical advances in the field of cardiology. These medicines are essential particularly for people who already have well-established disease. And again, it is the individual risk profile that will determine which medicines at which doses are most effective.

Sounds like a lot of work? Maybe. But remember: There is no immunity from heart disease. It potentially affects all of us. In fact, more people are disabled by heart disease than by all other medical problems combined! Learning the latest information about heart disease prevention means nothing less than insuring your own longevity and the longevity of your entire family.

Appendix:

Women and Estrogen— Yes or No?

Premenopausal women are at a much lower risk for heart disease than men the same age. This advantage disappears after menopause, and the reason is well known: After menopause, women stop producing estrogens. Estrogens have many functions, among them several that have a very positive effect on cardiac health. They change the number and character of LDL and HDL particles and exert a protective effect upon the endothelial cell lining the arterial wall. In addition, they facilitate relaxation of the coronary artery wall, allowing for increased blood flow and less plaque rupture.

When these effects of estrogen disappear after menopause, certain predictable things happen to a woman's risk factors. LDL particle distribution can profoundly change, resulting in a doubling in the number of women who are subclass B. Compounding this is a gradual rise in both LDL cholesterol levels and Apoprotein B concentrations. Rising Apoprotein B levels mean more LDL particles are forming in direct proportion to the increases in LDL cholesterol, thereby amplifying the LDL risk, even if the woman retains her original subclass A status. Women who change subclasses from A to B are catapulted into a super high risk category. While this is happening, HDL levels remain more or less flat. Unchanging HDLs in the face of substantially rising LDL cholesterol and the number of LDL particles means the reverse cholesterol transport system is failing.

For a woman to make an intelligent appraisal of her post-menopausal risk, she should re-examine the condition of her reverse cholesterol transport system. Her LDL status must be re-examined. First, recheck your basic lipid profile: HDL cholesterol, LDL cholesterol, triglycerides, total cholesterol, Apoprotein B, and LDL subclass. A rising Apoprotein B content out of proportion to the rise in LDL cholesterol is a tip-off that LDL subclass is changing. If the LDL subclass has changed, risk has increased by at least 300 percent. HDL subclass should be checked as well, to see if you are shifting to the less favorable HDL3 zone. The HDL status that conferred protection before menopause may now be gone.

These kinds of laboratory assessments have to be integrated into the woman's overall profile of other risks: diabetes, obesity, high blood pressure, smoking, family history. The presence of any of these other risk factors provides a compelling argument in favor of postmenopausal hormone therapy—if you're only considering the risk of heart disease. But there are other things to consider, and this is where decisions can become agonizing. Everything depends on weighing statistical risks, a concept not always easy to understand, and not always easy to act upon even when it is understood.

The risks of estrogen therapy are not to be underplayed and may be considered by many to be much worse than the risk of heart disease. The main risk of estrogen therapy is one of the most frightening diseases in all of medicine: cancer.

Breast Cancer

For women with no other risk factors for breast cancer, the exact magnitude of the increased risk of that disease represented by taking estrogen isn't clear, but there is increased risk. Even though the risk for heart disease is much greater in most women than the risk for breast cancer, it may be hard to consider such statistics coldly.

If menopause seriously changes your risk for heart disease in the ways described above, fear of breast cancer shouldn't keep you from considering the use of hormones. In the general population of women, the risk of developing coronary artery disease after age fifty is three to four times greater than the risk of developing breast cancer, and the risk of death from a heart attack is six times greater than the risk of death from breast cancer. These numbers do not of course apply to women who have known risks for breast cancer. Nor, on the other hand, do they apply to the women who have the greatest risk for heart disease. For instance, a woman who is subclass B with low HDL2 and high Lp(a)—not an uncommon combination—has sixteen times the average risk, a level that approaches certainty.

Increased Risk for Breast Cancer

- Prior cancer in other breast
- Family history
- Early menstruation (increased "estrogen time")
- Late menopause (increased "estrogen time")
- No pregnancies
- Obesity
- High-fat diet
- Estrogen use
- Alcohol

Decreased Risk for Breast Cancer

- Exercise
- Early pregnancy
- Low-fat, high-fiber diet

Certainly any woman with decreased breast cancer risk and increased heart disease risk should consider estrogen replacement therapy, as should anyone whose risk of breast cancer is neutral but whose risk of heart disease is very high. If you decide to use estrogen therapy, you should have a yearly mammogram.

Endometrial Cancer

The other specter is endometrial cancer. Here the discussion is a bit more complicated. This risk can be completely avoided by not taking pure estrogens—but pure estrogens are best for preventing heart disease. Estrogens (Premarin, Estratab, Ogen, Menest, Ortho-Est, Estropipate, Estrace, and Estraderm) can cause various kinds of precancerous changes in the lining of the uterus. This will occur in one out of three women taking pure estrogens for three years. That's a prohibitive statistic. If a woman has had a hysterectomy, there's no problem.

Women on estrogen therapy, therefore, require very close supervision by a gynecologist including yearly biopsies—not Pap smears—of their uterus. Obviously, you must have a very good reason to take pure estrogens if your uterus is intact.

Combination Therapy

The way around this dilemma is to take an estrogen combined with a progestin, the other female hormone that checks and balances the effects of estrogens. This will prevent the uterine abnormalities, although it may not be as effective as pure estrogen in reducing cardiac risks.

On average, pure estrogens will raise HDL cholesterol levels by about 7.5 mg. That's about the same as the exercise effect for accomplished long-distance runners. This response will occur after about six to twelve months of use. Estrogen-progestin combinations will yield less of an effect, with HDLs rising about 4.5—about the same as running twenty miles a week.

The effects on LDL cholesterol levels are not as pronounced, but they can be expected to fall by about 15 mgs in two to six months. What is more important is reconversion to subclass A from B, if this was a problem. This can be expected but shouldn't be taken for granted and must be checked.

The percentages of HDL2 can also be expected to be restored, even if HDL levels haven't changed much. And Lp(a) levels will fall. But estrogens cause triglycerides to rise slightly and should not be used if your initial triglyceride level is greater than 500.

One of the factors in the decision to use pure estrogen versus combination therapy will be the magnitude of the effect you want. If you have high LDLs and low HDLs then your risk profile can be an indication for pure estrogens. If combined hormone therapy is still chosen, it may require the addition of other lipid-lowering drugs.

Some anti–risk-factor medications can be avoided by taking estrogens, depending on which risks are being targeted:

Problem	Use Estrogen Replacement Instead of:
LDL subclass A, high LDL cholesterol	statins, resins
LDL subclass A, high Apoprotein B	statins, resins
LDL subclass B	niacin, resins
Low HDL cholesterol, low HDL2	niacin, fibrates
High Lp(a)	niacin
High fibrinogen	fibrates

Even when not dealing with extreme situations, estrogen is unlikely to be a cure-all. LDL cholesterol reductions are modest and often need supplementation with an anticholesterol drug. For subclass As, statins and estrogen are a very well tolerated combination. Estrogen, however, could be conceived as the "natural" first-line medication, which should be allowed about six months to reveal its effects.

Pills are more effective than patches, since pills are circulated from the intestines directly into the liver where the bulk of their effects take place. These hormones are taken in twenty-eight-day cycles, but the specific preparation and frequency best for you must be decided with your doctor.

The replacement therapy should begin as soon after menopause as possible. Duration of treatment is still a bit controversial, but the standard now is to continue therapy for at least ten years or until the midsixties. However, there is some strong evidence that older women still see benefits. Additionally, in older women, the protection against another scourge, osteoporosis, is lost if the drugs are stopped.

Other Factors

Finally, there are other noncardiac factors that must be weighed against one another in making the decision whether or not to take estrogen. Women with gallbladder disease, liver disease, clotting disorders, a history of phlebitis, migraines, or stroke should be wary and carefully discuss the matter with their doctors. Estrogens can aggravate these problems. On the other hand, osteoporosis, which can be a crippling problem later in life, responds well to estrogen therapy.

Estrogens are an elegant way of fighting heart disease. For most women, a careful weighing of the pros and cons with their doctors, and the proper follow-up afterward will ensure reaping the benefits and minimizing the risks.

Glossary

adrenalin A hormone secreted by the adrenal glands that stimulates heartbeat, raises blood pressure, and heightens mental alertness.

ALP Atherogenic lipoprotein profile.

anabolic steroids Hormones such as testosterone that simulate muscle tissue growth and male secondary sex characteristics.

angina Pain produced by the heart muscle in response to insufficient blood flow.

angiogram A study of the heart conducted by injecting dye into the coronary arteries.

angioplasty The mechanical removal of an atherosclerotic blockage or plaque by use of an inflated balloon introduced into the coronary artery by a catheter.

angstrom One ten-millionth of a millimeter.

aorta The body's largest artery into which the left ventricle of the heart empties.

aortic aneurysm A ballooning or bulging of the aorta caused by a weakening in the arterial wall.

Apo-A Apoprotein A.

Apo-B Apoprotein B.

Apo-E gene The actual sequence of protein bases on a chromosome that code for Apoprotein E.

Apo-E isoform A form of the Apoprotein E allele.

Apo-E Apoprotein E.

apoprotein Any of the many complex protein molecules that attach to the various lipid particles to form a lipoprotein.

Apoprotein A The protein attached to HDL particles that serves as an identifier, enzyme activator, and steering mechanism through the circulation.

Apoprotein B The protein attached to a variety of lipid particles, including LDL and VLDL particles, that acts as a steering mechanism through the circulation where it attaches to receptors at sites of lipid metabolism.

Apoprotein C-II   An apoprotein important in stimulating the reverse cholesterol transport reaction.

Apoprotein E   A protein attached to a variety of lipid particles, especially VLDLs, that interacts with cholesterol receptors essential to the processing of lipids by the liver.

Apoprotein E allele   One of the possible forms of the Apoprotein E gene. Each person has a set of two alleles, one from each parent.

atherogenic lipoprotein profile (ALP)   A combination of genes affecting metabolism and the generation of lipid particles that is responsible for the LDL subclass B state.

atherosclerosis   "Hardening of the arteries." The progressive accumulation of cholesterol, calcium, and blood clots on the wall of an artery.

atherosclerotic lesion   The lesion of arteriosclerosis, comprising highly variable proportions of cholesterol, calcium, immune cells, and clotted blood.

atrovastatin   Brand name Lipitor. A medication that reduces LDL cholesterol by reducing the number of subclass A particles.

beta-blocker cardiac medication   A medication that blocks the stimulatory properties of adrenalinelike hormones on the heart and blood vessels.

bile acid binding resins   A class of drugs that reduces cholesterol levels by blocking the reabsorption of cholesterol discarded by the liver into the intestines.

blood clot   A complex combination of platelets, clotting "fibers," and red blood cells that forms a solid or semisolid mass.

blood gas   A test that measures pH of the blood and its levels of oxygen and carbon dioxide.

BMI   body mass index.

body mass index   A measure of body size derived from weight and height measurements.

cardiovascular dysmetabolic syndrome (CDS)   A complex physiological-metabolic state manifested by high cholesterol, diabetes, and high blood pressure. Associated with subclass B lipid profiles and an extremely potent promoter of atherosclerosis.

cerebral vascular disease Abnormalities of the blood vessels supplying the brain. These are often related to atherosclerosis and are a cause of stroke.

cholesterol A lipid formed in the liver and other tissues from saturated fats and used in a multitude of important metabolic functions, including the production of hormones and the construction of cellular membranes. The molecule is always found in combination with proteins.

cholestyramine A bile acid binding resin.

chylomicrons Lipid particles that convey ingested and absorbed triglycerides from the intestines through the circulation. Most plentiful after a meal, they carry fat to the liver for metabolism and directly to other tissues prepared to utilize these fats.

claudication The interruption of nutrient arterial blood flow to a region of the body resulting in pain.

Colestid Colestipol. A bile acid binder.

coronary artery disease The atherosclerotic blockage of nutrient blood flow in the arteries of the heart resulting in pain and impairment of the heart muscle function.

Diabetes A multifaceted disease manifested by a disturbance in the normal relationship of blood sugar and insulin. High glucose levels in the blood are the result.

Echocardiogram A sonogram that studies the anatomy of the heart in movement.

EKG Electrocardiogram.

electrocardiogram A study of the electrical signals emitted by the contracting heart.

endothelial cells The cells that line the inner surface of the blood vessel and that are in direct contact with the bloodstream.

Estrace An estrogen derivative.

Estraderm An estrogen derivative.

Estratab An estrogen derivative.

estrogen A hormone that maintains female secondary sex characteristics and has significant impact on metabolism, including the metabolism and production of lipids.

Estropipate An estrogen derivative.

familial combined hyperlipidemia An inherited disorder produced by a multitude of genes in combination and characterized by very high levels of both LDL cholesterol, total cholesterol, and triglycerides. Also called "FCH."

familial hypercholesterolemia   An inherited disorder produced by a multitude of genes causing extreme elevations of total and LDL cholesterol. Also called "FH."

fasting blood sugar   Blood sugar level taken in the morning before eating and therefore reflective of one's baseline blood sugar level before interference by recently ingested food.

fasting insulin level   Insulin level taken in the morning before eating and therefore reflective of one's baseline insulin level before interference by recently ingested food.

fiber   A component of nonanimal food sources. Insoluble fibers are nondigestible components of plant cell walls and increase bowel motility. Soluble fibers are also derived from plant cell walls, but they dissolve to bind lipids in the intestine.

fibrates   Fibric acid derivative medications. These cause increased LPL activity, reduction of triglycerides and sometimes, reduction of LDL levels.

fibric acid derivatives   Fibrates.

fibrin   The end product of fibrinogen activation. The strandlike web or superstructure of a blood clot.

fibrinogen   The circulating clotting factor that, when activated, transforms into fibrin strands to trap blood cells and form the blood clot.

fibrinolysis   The lysis, or dissolution, of the strands of fibrin of a blood clot.

fibrosis   The replacement of living, metabolically active structural cells of any tissue with relatively inert and nonfunctional cells.

fissured plaque   An atherosclerotic plaque that has developed a crack in its surface.

foam cells   Originally normal immune cells that inhabit the inner layer of the arterial cell wall but have been stimulated to engulf large quantities of LDL and IDL particles.

folate   Folic acid, a B vitamin essential to normal metabolism.

genetic marker   Any detectable substance that is a manifestation of specific gene activity can be considered an indirect genetic marker. A specific gene known to cause or represent a specific trait or condition is a direct genetic marker.

glucose tolerance test   A repetitive hourly sampling of one's blood glucose level in response to ingestion of a standardized amount of sugar. A sensitive screening test for diabetes.

gradient gel electrophoresis   A blood test that sifts and identifies different elements of the blood by propelling the blood through a gel using an electric current.

HDL   High-density lipoprotein.

HDL cholesterol   The amount or blood concentration of cholesterol found attached to the high-density lipoprotein particle. The so-called good cholesterol.

HDL-GGE   HDL gradient gel electrophoresis

HDL subclass   The different types of HDL particles, as distinguished by gradient gel electrophoresis.

hemoglobin AC level   A measure of the amount of glucose attached to the hemoglobin molecule. This indicates the adequacy of blood glucose regulation by insulin.

high-density lipoprotein   The lipid particle responsible for reverse cholesterol transport. It contains cholesterol, triglycerides, and Apoprotein A.

homocysteine   A circulating amino acid that at abnormally elevated levels predisposes toward atherosclerosis by damaging endothelial cells and promoting blood clotting.

homocysteinemia   Abnormal elevation of blood homocysteine levels.

hypertriglyceridemia   Abnormal elevation of blood triglyceride levels.

Hypo A   Hypoapoprotein A. A genetic inability to produce HDL particles.

hypoalphalipoproteinemia   Hypo A.

Hypoapoprotein A   A genetic disorder manifested by low HDL levels caused by an intrinsic inability to produce HDL particles. The confirmatory test is the measurement of Apoprotein A levels, which will be low.

ICU   Intensive care unit.

IDL   Intermediate-density lipoprotein.

intermediate-density lipoprotein   A major carrier of cholesterol in the blood.

immune scavenger cells   White blood cells, tissue repair cells, and other cell types whose function is to eliminate foreign substances in any area of the body.

infarction   The death of living tissue resulting from interruption of nutrient blood flow.

insulin   The regulatory hormone secreted by the pancreas that modulates blood glucose levels, allows glucose to penetrate cell membranes that require it for food, and modulates fat metabolism and the production of lipid particles.

intrinsic fibrinolysis   The body's ability to dissolve its own blood clots without the administration of drugs.

LDL cholesterol   The amount or blood concentration of cholesterol found attached to the low-density lipoprotein particle.

LDL cholesterol particle   A particle containing cholesterol, triglyceride, and an Apoprotein B. The single greatest metabolic risk factor for atherosclerosis. These particles come in at least seven different sizes and densities.

LDL   Low-density lipoprotein.

LDL-GGE   LDL gradient gel electrophoresis.

LDL subclass   The family of LDL particles a particular LDL particle belongs to as determined by its size and density.

LDL subclass A   The family of LDL particles of relatively low density and larger size.

LDL subclass B   The family of LDL particles of relatively high density and smaller size.

lipids   A broad class of compounds including fatty acids and cholesterol characterized by long chains of carbon atoms. In medicine, the term is used to refer to circulating lipid-containing particles: VLDL, IDL, LDL, HDL, triglycerides, Lp(a).

Lipitor   Brand name of atrovastatin.

Lipoprotein a   Lp(a). An LDL particle attached to an apoprotein A. The combination is genetically determined and is a risk factor for heart disease.

lipoprotein lipase   A family of enzymes crucial in the metabolism of fatty acids from triglycerides. Plays a key role in mediating the effects of exercise on lipid metabolism.

lovastatin   A statin drug.

Low-density lipoprotein cholesterol   The cholesterol quantity found attached to LDL particles. The so-called bad cholesterol.

Lp(a)   Lipoprotein a.

LPL   Lipoprotein lipase.

Menest   Brand name for an estrogen derivative.

metabolic risk factor   A risk factor for coronary disease that is the result of the metabolism of lipids and that circulates at certain levels in the blood.

Mevacor   Brand name of Lovastatin.

monounsaturated fat   A form of naturally occurring fat that has a chain of carbon atoms, all but one of which are linked by an unsaturated (nonhydrogenated) bond.

niacin   B vitamin intimately involved with energy metabolism. In the form of nicotinic acid, it acts to inhibit cholesterol synthesis, to increase cholesterol disposal, and to reduce triglyceride levels.

Ogen   Brand name for an estrogen derivative.

omega fatty acid   Omega-6 and omega-3 polyunsaturated fatty acids. The number designation refers to the point in the carbon chain where the carbon bond is saturated, the other bonds being unsaturated. Omega-3 fats are mainly found in marine animals and omega 6 in vegetable oils.

Ortho-Est   Brand name for an estrogen derivative.

osteoporosis   The gradual decalcification and weakening of the bones with age, prolonged illness, or hormonal changes.

oxidation   The combination of oxygen with other molecules or the loss of electrons by one molecule to another. In the natural systems discussed in this book, the oxidation effect results in a net destabilization of any system by making it more chemically reactive to its microenvironment.

oxidized LDL particles   LDL particles whose surface layer of molecules have been made more chemically reactive by being exposed to an oxidizing agent.

peripheral vascular disease   Atherosclerotic blockages and impaired blood flow in arteries supplying the extremities.

phlebitis   An inflammation of the veins that may also involve the development of blood clots.

plaque   The lesion of atherosclerosis.

plaque rupture   The cracking of an atherosclerotic plaque often occurring at the point of adherence onto the blood vessel wall, allowing it to swing freely into the lumen of the blood vessel and stimulate blood clot formation.

plasminogen   The circulating blood factor that transforms into the clot-dissolving chemical called plasmin.

platelet   A circulating blood factor that is the first element of the blood clot.

polyunsaturated fat   A fatty acid that has more than one unhydrogenated carbon-carbon bond.

Pravachol   Brand name of pravastatin.

pravastatin   A statin drug.

Premarin   Brand name for an estrogen derivative.

progesterone   A hormone involved with pregnancy and the regulation of the menstrual cycle. It is also involved in the metabolism of lipids.

progestin   A progesterone derivative.

Questran   Brand name of cholestyramine.

reverse cholesterol transport   The uptake of cholesterol from the atherosclerotic lesion by HDL particles and its delivery for disposal by the liver and other agents.

risk profile   The individual's set of circulating risk factors for atherosclerosis.

Scavenger cells   Immune cells circulating in the blood and residing in tissues.

simvastatin   A statin drug.

statin   Informal name for a group of similar cholesterol-lowering drugs called HMG coenzyme A reductase inhibitors. These block the enzyme that produces cholesterol.

synergistic   The enhancement or amplification of a biological phenomenon by two or more concurring factors.

systolic blood pressure   The pressure the blood generates at the peak of heart constriction. The higher number in a blood pressure reading.

TC/HDL ratio   Total cholesterol/high density cholesterol ratio.

testosterone   The hormone responsible for male secondary sex characteristics.

TIA   Transient ischemic attack.

total cholesterol   The amount or concentration of cholesterol contained in all the various lipid particles as measured per unit of blood.

total cholesterol/high-density cholesterol ratio   A sensitive measure of heart disease risk arrived at by dividing the total cholesterol level by the HDL cholesterol level. The ratio should be below 4.

trans-fats Polyunsaturated fats whose geometric structures have been "bent" and partially hydrogenated, usually as a result of heating.

transient ischemic attack A temporary loss of function of part of the brain resulting from insufficient blood flow.

triglycerides The binding of three fatty acids to a glycerol molecule. This is the main form of naturally occurring fats both in the circulating blood and in storage in the cells.

two-hour postprandial blood sugar A blood sugar level taken two hours after a meal. Used as a screen for diabetes.

ventricle The main pumping chamber of the heart. The right ventricle pumps blood into the lung. The left ventricle pumps blood out to the body.

very low density lipoprotein VLDL. Lipid particle that is a precursor of the smaller IDLs and LDLs. They are the main carriers of triglycerides from the liver.

vitamin C Ascorbic acid. An essential component of many metabolic energy pathways. Essential in tissue repair and resistance to injury including oxidative stress. Also protects vitamin E from oxidation.

vitamin E A group of compounds called tocopherols most concentrated in vegetable oils. They act as stabilizing agents protecting the surfaces of lipid particles from oxidation.

VLDL Very low density lipoprotein.

Zocor Brand name of simvastatin.

Sources

Normal Lipid Levels in the Population

Brown et al. Plasma Lipid, Lipoprotein Cholesterol, and Apoprotein Distributions in Selected U.S. Communities, The Atherosclerosis Risk in Communities (ARIC) Study. *Arteriosclerosis and Thrombosis* 1993; 13: 1139–158.

> Probably the most comprehensive compilation of the normal distribution of lab values for most of the risk factors presented in this book divided according to age, sex, and race. This study is excellent for displaying trends with age.

Development of Atherosclerosis in the Young

Joseph et al. Manifestations of Coronary Atherosclerosis in Young Trauma Victims—An Autopsy Study. *Journal of the American College of Cardiology* 1993; 22: 459–67.

Stary. Evolution and Progression of Atherosclerotic Lesions in Coronary Arteries of Children and Young Adults. *Arteriosclerosis* Sup. I, 1989; 9: 1–19, 1–32.

Strong. Natural History and Risk Factors in Early Human Atherogenesis (The Pathobiological Determinants of Atherosclerosis in Youth—PDAY). *Clinical Chemistry* 1995; 41: 134–38.

The Behavior of Atherosclerotic Lesions

Fuster, Lewis A. Conner Memorial Lecture: Mechanisms Leading to Myocardial Infarction: Insights from Studies of Vascular Biology. *Circulation* 1994; 90: 2126–146.

————. Pathogenesis of Coronary Artery Disease: Biologic Role of Risk Factors. *Journal of American College of Cardiology* 1996; 27: 964–76.

Pusternak. The Spectrum of Risk Factors for Coronary Heart Disease. *Journal of American College of Cardiology* 1996; 27: 978–89.

Cholesterol Values in People with and without Heart Disease

Kannel. Range of Serum Cholesterol Values in the Population Developing Coronary Artery Disease. *American Journal of Cardiology* 1995; 76: 690–770.

Martin et al. Serum Cholesterol, Blood Pressure, and Mortality: Implications from a Cohort of 361,662 Men. *Lancet* 1986; 2: 933–36.

Wilson, Garrison, et al. Prevalence of Coronary Heart Disease in the Framingham Offspring Study: Role of Lipoprotein Cholesterols. *American Journal of Cardiology* 1980; 46: 649–54.

Genetic Influences

Genest et al. Familial Lipoprotein Disorders in Patients with Premature Coronary Artery Disease. *Circulation* 1992; 85: 2025–033.

Genetics and Environmental Contributions to Cardiovascular Risk Factors in Mexican Americans—The San Antonio Family Heart Study, *Circulation* 1996; 94: 2159–170.

LDL Cholesterol Reduction and Prevention, Control and Regression of Coronary Artery Disease including the Different Effects of Medications

Helsinki Heart Study

Blankenhorn et al. CLAS: Beneficial Effects of Combined Colestipol-Niacin Therapy on Coronary Atherosclerosis and Coronary Venous Bypass Grafts. *JAMA* 1987; 257: 3233–240.
  Actually showed by coronary angiography what the Helsinki Study implied: actual melting of coronary lesions in response

to therapy by people with low HDL and high triglycerides regardless of LDL levels.

Manninen et al. The Helsinki Heart Study: Joint Effects of Serum Triglyceride and LDL Cholesterol and HDL Cholesterol Concentrations on Coronary Artery Disease Risk in the Helsinki Heart Study. *Circulation,* June 1992; 85: 37–45.

The only people who benefited from a fibrate drug were the ones who had elevated triglycerides and low HDL levels regardless of their LDL cholesterol level.

National Heart, Lung, and Blood Institute Study

Brensike et al. (NHLBI type II) National Heart, Lung and Blood Institute type II Trial: The Influences of Changes in Lipid Values Induced by Cholestyramine and Diet on Progression of Coronary Artery Disease. *Circulation* 1984; 69: 325–37.

Using coronary angiograms revealed the IDL-LDL subclass connection by showing that the people whose atherosclerosis melted had reduction of intermediate density (IDL) and small, dense LDL particle types.

The Familial Atherosclerosis Treatment Study

Brown et al. The Familial Atherosclerosis Treatment Study Series (FATS): Regression of Coronary Artery Disease as a Result of Intensive Lipid Lowering Therapy in Men with High Levels of ApoB. *New England Journal of Medicine* Nov. 1990; 323: 1289–298.

Stewart et al. Benefits of Lipid Lowering Therapy in Men with Elevated ApoB Not Confined to Those with Very High LDL. *Journal of American College of Cardiology* 1994; 23: 899–906.

Hepatic Lipase Changes Predicts Coronary Artery Disease Regression/Progression in FATS. *Circulation* 1996; 94: I539.

In a group of relatively young men with strong family histories of heart disease, the predominance of LDL subclass B was identified as the major risk factor at any level of LDL. People with subclass B starting at relatively low LDL levels demonstrated more melting of lesions in response to appropriate treatments than subclass As enjoying much greater levels of LDL reduction.

MARS (Monitored Atherosclerosis Regression Study)

Blankenhorn et al. Coronary Angiographic Changes with Lova-statin Therapy—the MARS Study. *Annals of Internal Medicine* 1993; 119: 969–76.

Hodis et al. Triglyceride and Cholesterol Rich Lipoproteins Have a Differential Effect on Mild/Moderate and Severe Lesion Progression as Assessed by Quantitative Coronary Angiography in a Controlled Trial of Lovastatin. *Circulation* 1994; 90: 42–49.

Mack et al. Lipoprotein Subclasses in (MARS), *Arteriosclerosis Thrombosis. Vascular Biology* 1996; 16: 697–704.
> Demonstrated the differential risk factor sensitivities of old ver-sus young coronary artery lesions and the sensitivity of the dis-ease progression in low LDL cholesterol people with triglyc-eride rich (subclass B–type) lipoproteins.

STARS (Saint Thomas's Atherosclerosis Regression Study)

Watts et al. Effects on Coronary Artery Disease of Lipid Lower-ing Diet, or Diet Plus Cholestyramine, in St. Thomas' Athero-sclerosis Regression Study. *Lancet,* 339: 563–69.

———. Independent Associations between Plasma Lipoprotein Subfraction Levels and the Course of CAD in STARS. *Metabolism* 1993; 42: 1461–67.

SCRIPT (The Stanford Coronary Risk Intervention Project)

Haskell et al. Effects of Intensive Multiple Risk Factor Reduction on Coronary Atherosclerosis and Clinical Cardiac Events in Men and Women with Coronary Artery Disease—The Stanford Coronary Risk Intervention Project. *Circulation* 1994; 89: 975–90.

Miller et al. Predominance of Dense Low Density Lipoprotein Particles Predicts Angiographic Benefit of Therapy in SCRIPT. *Circulation* 1996; 94: 2146–153.
> These sets of studies confirmed that subclass B particle levels were most closely associated with growth of coronary artery lesions.

LDL Reduction with Statins

Pedersen et al. Cholesterol Lowering and the Use of Healthcare Resources—Results of the Scandinavian Simvastatin Survival Study. *Circulation* 1996; 93: 1796–802.

Sacks et al. The Effect of Provastatin on Coronary Events after Myocardial Infarction in Patients with Average Cholesterol Levels. *New England Journal of Medicine* 1996; 335: 1001–1009.

Shepherd et al. Prevention of CAD with Pravastatin in Men with Hypercholesterolemia. *New England Journal of Medicine* 1995; 333: 1301–307.

This set of studies confirmed the importance of reducing LDL cholesterol levels in all people: people with and without coronary artery disease and people with and without "elevated" LDL levels. Subclasses were not differentiated. People with average cholesterol levels benefit from further reductions.

Lewis et al. Effect of Pravastatin on Cardiovascular Events in Women after Myocardial Infarction: the CARE Trial. *Journal of American College of Cardiology* 1998; 32: 140–46.

Superko. Lipid Disorders Contributing to Coronary Artery Disease: An Update. *Current Problems in Cardiology* Nov. 1996; 21: 736–80.

A comprehensive review of the above studies and the medication-treatment implications. The single best discussion of the topic.

Studies Demonstrating the Specific Impact of LDL Subclass B on Coronary Artery Disease

Gardner et al. Association of Small-Density Lipoprotein Particles with the Incidence of Coronary Artery Disease in Men and Women. *JAMA* 1996; 276: 875–81.

Lamarche et al. Small, Dense Low Density Lipoprotein Particles as a Predictor of the Risk of Ischemic Heart Disease in Men—Quebec Cardiovascular Study. *Circulation* 1997; 95: 69–75.

Stumpfor et al. A Prospective Study of Triglyceride Level, Low Density Lipoprotein Particle Diameter, and Risk of Myocardial Infarction. *JAMA* 1996; 276: 882–88.

Tornvall et al. Relation of Plasma Levels and Composition of Apolipoprotein B–Containing Lipoproteins to Angiographically Defined Coronary Artery Disease in Young Patients with Myocardial Infarction. *Circulation* 1993; 88: 2180–189.
Key article demonstrating significance of subclass B particles and premature coronary artery disease.

Relationship of Subclass B to Other Lipid Variables

Austin et al. Atherogenic Lipoprotein Phenotype, A Proposed Genetic Marker for Coronary Artery Disease Risk. *Circulation* 1990; 82: 495–506.

Krauss. Heterogeneity of Plasma Low Density Lipoproteins and Atherosclerosis Risk, *Current Opinion in Lipidology* 1994; 5: 339–49.

HDL

Buring et al. Decreased HDL2 and HDL3 Cholesterol, Apo A-1 and Apo A-II, and Increased Risk of Myocardial Infarction. *Circulation* 1992; 85: 22–29.

Salomen et al. HDL1, HDL2, and HDL3 Subfractions and the Risk of Acute Myocardial Infarction. A Prospective Population Study in Eastern Finnish Men. *Circulation* 1991; 84: 129–39.

Williams. Effects of Weight Loss by Exercise or Diet on Plasma HDL Levels in Men with Low, Intermediate and Normal to High HDL at Baseline. *Metabolism* 1994; 43: 912–24.

Blood Clotting and Other Risk Factors

Ridker. Beyond Cholesterol: Novel Risk Factors for Atherosclerotic Disease. *Cardiology Rounds* 1997; 1: no. 1.
A good overall review of clotting factors, Lp(a), and homocysteine with a good bibliography for reference.

Exercise

Coyle. Fat Metabolism during Exercise (a Review), Sports Nutrition Workshop. *Sports Science Exchange* 1995; 8: no. 6.

Despres and Lamarche. Low-Intensity Endurance Exercise Training, Plasma Lipoproteins and the Risk of Coronary Heart Disease. *Journal of Internal Medicine* 1994; 236.
    Elaborates the idea of "metabolic fitness."

Hambrecht et al. Various Intensities of Leisure Time Physical Activity in Patients with Coronary Artery Disease. *Journal American College of Cardiology* 1993; 22: 468–77.
    Demonstration by angiography of exercise threshold responses in coronary artery lesions.

Wood. Physical Activity, Diet, and Health Independent and Interactive Effects. *Medicine and Science in Sports and Exercise* 1994; 26: 838–40.

Senti et al. Long Term Physical Exercise and Quantitatively Assessed Human Coronary Collateral Circulation. *Journal of American College of Cardiology* 1998; 32: 49–56.
    Shows association between amount of exercise performed and re-routing of blood flow to circumvent blocked coronary arteries. Good current bibliography on topic.

Superko. Exercise Training, Serum Lipids, and Lipoprotein Particles: Is There a Change Threshold? *Medicine and Science in Sports and Exercise* 1991; 23: 677–80.

Williams. Relationship of Distance Run Per Week to Coronary Artery Disease Risk Factors in 8283 Male Runners—The National Runners' Health Study. *Arch Internal Medicine* 1997; 157: 191–98.

Diet and Weight Loss

Chait et al. Rationale of the Diet—Heart Statement of the American Heart Association—Report of the Nutrition Committee. *Circulation* 1993; 88: 3009–029.

Dreon et al. Apoprotein E Isoform Phenotype and LDL Subclass Response to a Reduced Fat Diet. *Arteriosclerosis Thrombosis Vascular Biology* 1995; 15: 105–11.

————. LDL Subclass Patterns and Lipoprotein Response to a Low Fat, High Carbohydrate Diet in Women. *Arteriosclerosis Thrombosis Vascular Biology* 1997; 17: 707–14.

Krauss and Dreon. Low Density Lipoprotein Subclasses and Response to a Low-Fat Diet in Healthy Men. *American Journal of Clinical Nutrition* 1995; 62: 478–87S.

Williams et al. Effects of Dietary Fat on HDL Subclasses Are Influenced by Both ApoE Isoforms and LDL Subclass Patterns. *American Journal of Clinical Nutrition* 1995; 61: 1234–40.

Index